Medical Humanities Companion

VOLUME FOUR

Medical Humanities Companion
VOLUME FOUR

Prognosis

Edited by
Jill Gordon
Jane Macnaughton
and
Carl Edvard Rudebeck

Series Editors
Rolf Ahlzén, Martyn Evans, Pekka Louhiala
and Raimo Puustinen

Radcliffe Publishing
Oxford • New York

Radcliffe Publishing Ltd
St Mark's House
Shepherdess Walk
London
N1 7LH
United Kingdom

www.radcliffehealth.com

Electronic catalogue and worldwide online ordering facility.

British Library Cataloguing in Publication Data

A catalogue record for this book is available from the British Library.

ISBN-13: 978 184619 555 6

Typeset by Phoenix Photosetting, Chatham, Kent, UK
Printed and bound by Cadmus Communications, USA

Contents

About the editors and authors

Rolf Ahlzén is a general practitioner and an assistant professor in medical humanities at Karlstad University in Sweden. He has an academic background both in the humanities and in medicine, and he is the chairman of the Regional Ethical Committee.

Martyn Evans is Professor of Humanities in Medicine at Durham University, and Principal of Trevelyan College. He was founding joint editor of the Medical Humanities edition of the Journal of Medical Ethics from 2000 to 2008. He has published variously on the aesthetics of music, ethics and philosophy of medicine, the role of humanities in medical education, music and medicine and the philosophy of wonder in relation to medicine. In 2005 he was made an honorary Fellow of the Royal College of General Practitioners.

Jill Gordon is a general practitioner specialising in psychotherapy in primary care in Sydney. She is President of the Australian College of Psychological Medicine and an honorary professor at the University of Sydney where she initiated Australia's first postgraduate degree in medical humanities.

Iona Heath worked as a GP in Kentish Town in London from 1975 to 2010. She was President of the Royal College of General Practitioners, UK, from 2009 to 2012.

Pekka Louhiala is a lecturer in medical ethics at the University of Helsinki, Finland. He has degrees in both medicine and philosophy, and he also works as a part-time paediatrician in private practice. He has published on various topics in medical ethics, philosophy of medicine and epidemiology. His current academic interests include conceptual and philosophical issues in medicine, such as evidence-based medicine and placebo effects.

Anne Macleod, poet and novelist, was formerly Associate Specialist in Dermatology at Aberdeen Royal Infirmary.

Jane Macnaughton is Professor of Medical Humanities and Co-Director of the Centre for Medical Humanities at Durham University. She is also Deputy Head of the University's School of Medicine and Health and teaches on its undergraduate medical programme. She has published on a wide range of themes within the medical humanities, including the doctor–patient relationship, embodied practice, medical education and the role of medical humanities in critiquing the evidence-base of biomedicine. Having worked as a GP before moving to full time academic work in Durham, Jane now does part-time clinical work in gynaecology and is Honorary Consultant in Obstetrics and Gynaecology at the University Hospital of North Durham.

Raimo Puustinen is a general practitioner with 30 years of clinical experience. He currently works as an acting professor of General Practice at the University of Tampere Medical School, Finland. He has published articles and books on general practice, medical ethics and philosophy of medicine. When not practising medicine or contemplating theoretical issues in medical practice, he plays jazz on the tenor saxophone and blues with a blues harp. He is married, and has four children and six grandchildren.

Carl Edvard Rudebeck is a general practitioner from Västervik in Sweden. He is a research advisor in the healthcare organisation of Kalmar county, and part-time professor of general practice at Tromsö University in Norway. He is involved in various qualitative research projects in general practice and physiotherapy. He has put much interest into the theoretical aspects of general practice as a discipline, and into the phenomenology of body experience and the phenomenology of the doctor–patient interaction.

John Saunders is a consultant physician in Abergavenny, South Wales; honorary professor at Swansea University; former visiting professor at the University of Otago, New Zealand; and honorary senior lecturer at Cardiff University. He was formerly an associate editor of *Medical Humanities*, chair of the Research Ethics Committee for Wales; and is current chair of ethics at the Royal College of Physicians. He recently completed postgraduate studies in philosophy at University College London.

Acknowledgements

As always, we are grateful to Gillian Nineham, the Editorial Director at Radcliffe Publishing, for her encouragement throughout the publication of the four volumes in the series, and to the editorial staff.

We have made it a tradition to meet each year to discuss our respective contributions to each volume. Our meeting in Helsinki, Finland in 2012 was organised by our fellow writer Pekka Louhiala and was supported by the Signe and Ane Gyllenberg Foundation.

During our visit we were honoured to present a seminar on the humanities in medicine with additional support from two graduate schools at the University of Helsinki: Doctoral Programs in Public Health and the National Graduate School for Clinical Science. Their support is also acknowledged with thanks. The seminar was opened by Raimo Puustinen and the papers presented were 'What is Medical Humanities?' (Martyn Evans), 'Why Medical Humanities? Applications in General Practice' (Iona Heath), 'Medical Humanities and Clinical Research' (John Saunders), 'Medical Humanities and the Clinical Encounter' (Jill Gordon), 'Why Should Physicians Read?' (Rolf Ahlzén), 'Hermeneutics and Clinical Understanding' (Carl Edvard Rudebeck) and 'Research in Medical Humanities' (Jane Macnaughton).

We stayed in the Hanasaari Hanaholmen Hotel in a serene location on the Hanasaari Peninsula between Espoo and Helsinki. The hotel is part of a cultural centre that promotes cooperation and exchange between Finland and Sweden, and it certainly promoted cooperation between members of our group, not only our Finnish and Swedish colleagues! We acknowledge one another as critical friends in the writing process.

Introduction

We began our *Companion* series with stories of everyday people and everyday illnesses. We met Rachel, Jake, Liz, Geoff and Jen in stories woven by our virtual writer in residence, dermatologist Anne MacLeod.* Although Anne created the characters in the *Companion* series along with their illnesses and their illness progression, each of us cannot help but think about real people just like them, drawn from our own practices.

These stories have helped us, as a group of writers located in different parts of the world, to find particular threads in the stories and to follow them towards a better understanding of what it means to experience a symptom, receive a diagnosis or undergo treatment.

While writing the chapters for each volume, we have met once a year and have been privileged to be able to exchange ideas, squabble, laugh, expostulate and support one another in our agreed tasks. We have met in Italy, England, Sweden, Scotland and Finland. (Despite encouragement from one of the editors of this present volume, we have not quite managed to meet in Australia – yet.) Emerging from these meetings and conversations is a heartening solidarity in our views about what really matters in the space between the patient and the doctor.

In Volume one, *Symptom*, we explored the significance of the transition from unthinking good health to awareness of the possibility that we may be ill. We put forward the claim that 'the notion of a symptom is as good a starting point as any for trying to take seriously the extraordinary fusion of the material and the existential that is conscious human experience'.

In Volume two, *Diagnosis*, we considered the idea that diagnoses 'shape and are shaped by our views on what is real, what is acceptable and how we relate to certain phenomena. Diagnoses are born and they die in a complex interaction between scientific discoveries, social negotiation and historical change'.

---

*   Anne lives near Inverness in Scotland. She has published two collections of poetry: *Standing By Thistles* (1997) and *Just The Caravaggio (1999)*. Anne has also published two novels: *The Dark Ship* (2002) and *The Blue Moon Book (2004)*.

Volume three, *Treatment*, turned us to the questions that arise when we start to interfere with the natural course of life events. Beauchamp and Childress[1] sum up the doctor's tasks with four pithy injunctions: nonmaleficence, beneficence, respect for autonomy and justice. In other words, 'Do no harm'; 'Try to do good'; 'Help your patient to realise his or her full potential'; and 'Oh, and by the way, remember that resources are limited and must be distributed as fairly as possible.' No wonder treatment is such a challenge.

Each of the volumes to date has drawn on our different perspectives on the humanities as they relate to medicine. These perspectives are essential to our understanding of what really goes on in the clinical encounter; without those ways of seeing, we are, all of us, impoverished.

In Act 1, Scene 4 of *The Tempest*, Prospero says that 'we are such stuff as dreams are made on and our little lives are rounded with a sleep,' and so it is that this fourth volume in our *Medical Humanities Companions* series points us in the direction of that rounding sleep. We come to grips with the challenge of the prognosis, of looking ahead, wondering about what will happen and trying to make sense of life and death. We're still focusing on Rachel, Jake, Liz, Geoff and Jen, but, as you will see in Chapter 1, time has moved on, and Geoff and Jen have both died. Rachel is reaching adulthood. Jake is reflecting on lost opportunities. Liz is reinventing herself with new possibilities. How often do we catch up with patients after an absence and find that they have gone down the exact path that we would have predicted? How often do we catch up with them and find that their lives have changed in surprising ways that we would never have predicted for them?

Imagine if our lives lacked the richness of that unpredictability. Imagine if prognosis were just a matter of entering data into a 'prognostication machine'. (Let's face it, that's what countless patients currently do with Dr Google.) Under those circumstances, our patients may simply enter their symptoms and their history, and bring the data to their consultation. The doctor could then add more data from the physical examination and test results.

The prognostication machine would have some definite advantages: it could provide an extensive written report for the patient to take home to read and re-read and to discuss with family. We all have patients who appreciate the annual 'executive health checks' that their firms require. We bite our collective tongues when it comes to judging the relevance of some of the information, but that is neither here nor there. Having a hard copy of all the information and its prognostic significance at least enables stressed executives to take their own time to adjust to its content and to decide whether and how to follow the inevitable recommendations for a healthier lifestyle.

What would the report from the prognostication machine lack? The answer to this question is really the *raison d'être* for this volume. As with our first volume, in which Martyn Evans vividly describes the symptoms of pneumonia, we start with Raimo Puustinen's personal experience of a potentially life-limiting prognosis. Raimo's story is that of so many of our patients, whose illness journey takes them far into the future, 'planning their own funerals' before their first medical consultation.

> The moment I heard my colleague's voice I knew there was something seriously wrong with my skin. And not just my skin, but my whole body, and eventually my whole existence.

This is *prognosis-as-lived* as Rolf Ahlzén calls it in Chapter 3. It is not simply an illness experience, but a 'whole of body, whole of existence' experience. As unique and as incommunicable as it may be, the ill person's perspective on their prognosis calls upon the attending and attentive physician, in the inter-subjective space of the consultation, to offer interpretation, explanation, judgement, wisdom and constancy.

Carl Edvard Rudebeck considers the connection between the ideas of time and commitment. The patient's initial presentation marks the beginning of a relationship and a mutual commitment to see the process through to its end. The commitment may involve risk and pain for both patient and doctor, because the relationship goes beyond the immediate biomedical facts of illness and treatment towards meaning and significance at each stage of the patient's life, even towards death.

Taking up another major theme of this volume and of the series, John Saunders discusses how medicine's success at abolishing many of the old causes of premature death has led to the possibility of a long life with chronic illness. His focus is on the ways in which this fact challenges the ideas of patient and doctor as lay person and expert. In a partnership, both contribute complementary knowledge of the disease and its prognosis, and share responsibility and commitment in its management. Even when the doctor is unable to exercise medical magic and make it all go away, he or she must bear witness to suffering, and foster a life of self-fulfilment and happiness within the context of illness. We need to know how to 'put the body in its place' since it is only one small determinant of the good life.

John's lead is taken up in the theme of 'becoming' in Chapter 6, where Jane Macnaughton examines how such flourishing can occur in the context of illness, even when it is severe, chronic or life limiting. Jane starts from a position that illness involves adaptation that may resemble, but be accelerated and be more intense than the adaptations that are a part of normal ageing. Human beings adapt to new becomings that have the potential to release extraordinary creativity and achievement. We must learn not to confine patients' own prognostic expectations within a narrow medical model.

There are other ways of dealing with a grim prognosis. In Chapter 7, Jill Gordon reflects on the conflict between dry, rational science and lively, irrational hope. Faced with a life-threatening prognosis it is tempting to seek the miracle cure that offers hope, no matter how tenuous, for longer life. Patients and their families can turn a tentative prognosis into a firm prediction – a prophecy, but the decision to do so comes at a cost. In Chapter 8, Pekka Louhiala illustrates why the idea of commitment is so crucial to good medical care. The relationship that leads to insight into the patient's personal perspective acts as a corrective to over-medicalisation – the application of unnecessary or potentially harmful treatment that may ignore the patient's values and desires. In Chapter 9, Iona Heath takes up these themes of time, commitment and the avoidance of harm in relation to the care of patients living through into old age. She challenges those who pay narrow, focused, attention to what medicine is capable of doing and implores us to consider instead what medical care should be doing.

Our themes of time, mutual commitment, change, becoming, hope and expectation for the future come together in Martyn Evans's final chapter 'Open futures, human finitude'. We all know the importance of living in the present, but we cannot help but imagine the future, and our presence within it. As our bodies start to show signs of age and illness, we have to contemplate the idea of not being, or some sense of being other than the physical or conscious. In an exploration of the noumenal, Martyn asks us to think about our experience as creatures who struggle to contemplate our own non-being and speculate on the unknowable future. Music exists in time and time in music but as Iain McGilchrist points out:

> Music does not so much free time from temporality as bring out an aspect that is always present within time, its intersection with a moment which partakes of eternity. Similarly it does not so much use the physical to transcend physicality, or use particularity to transcend the particular, as bring out the spirituality latent in what we conceive as physical existence and uncover the universality that is, as Goethe spent a lifetime trying to express, always latent in the particular.[2]

This volume ends, as the series began, with music, and music begins and ends in silence, just as conscious life does. A child emerges from eternity, takes a first breath, and cries. With any luck it will be many years before the silence falls again. Scientific medicine can only partly fathom the music within each life, but when the doctor listens and engages with that special attention born of both expertise and commitment, the consultation creates a space that allows medical care to achieve its true purpose and potential.

REFERENCES

1. Beauchamp TL and Childress JF. *Principles Of Biomedical Ethics.* 6th ed. Oxford: Oxford University Press; 2009.
2. McGilchrist I. *The Master and His Emissary: the divided brain and the making of the Western world.* New Haven, CT: Yale University Press; 2009. p. 77.

Narratives

ANNE MACLEOD

RACHEL: 15 YEARS OLD

Rachel presses her face against the rain-splattered window. Outside, it's already dark. A wind has got up, harrying the last of the autumn leaves. The trees are bare. Skeletal. 'Your mother's here.' Rachel says nothing. 'You can go home now, Rachel. It's time.' She turns at last. The nurse rattles the screen back, forcing a full view of the stripped-down bed across the room. 'Your prescription.' Rachel ignores the over-filled paper bag. She nods at the naked mattress.

'She OK?'

'She's in High Dependency.'

'But she'll get better, right?'

'Time will tell.' The nurse will not say more and she will not look Rachel in the eye. She sweeps from the room, leaving Rachel no alternative but to follow.

Her mother is standing at the end of the ward, murmuring to the charge nurse, their heads close together. As Rachel draws near, they fall silent and draw apart. Her mother's eyes are puffy, like she's been crying. 'Did Staff nurse talk you through the new insulin dose?' The charge nurse looks at Rachel naturally, as if nothing has happened.

'Yeah,' Rachel lies, sauntering through the doors and out of the ward, without acknowledging her mother. Not until she reaches the outer door does she stop walking.

The weather balks her and pins her on the step. She crouches on the cold stone, shivering. Rocking. And the memories flood back, too clear. High definition. She'd been off her head for weeks, careless with her insulin, not paying any attention to the flu, to the chest infection. *Why should she? Why did she have to be different?* And it wasn't good anyway, flaunting needles in front of Ollie and the others. They were always after needles. Which one of them had seen her pass out and phoned the ambulance? Not Ollie, she'd bet. Not Leila.

She remembered drifting in and out of consciousness. And then waking in that room, tied to an intravenous stand. Hadn't she always hated being tied down? First thing she did was pull the drip out.

'What you doing?' A voice from the next bed startled her.

'Duh? What's it look like?' Blood oozed across the white duvet, pooling in the hollows. There was nothing to press against her arm – no tissues, nothing. Across the room the girl flinched. Her hair was plastered to her head and her brown skin looked pale.

'You OK?' Rachel glowered.

'Pain in my belly.'

'Ain't they given you nothing for it?'

'Nurse said she'd come back. With an injection.'

'Lucky you.' Rachel found a towel at last, wrapped it around her arm and eased herself off the bed.

'Where you off to?'

'Where d' you think? The loo.'

'Better not let them … catch … you.' It clearly exhausted this girl just to talk.

'What's your name anyway?'

'Rachelle,' the girl whispered. 'But they don't get it right; they all call me Rachel.'

'They would. They're dumb.'

'What's your name?'

'Funnily enough it's Rachel. Cool to meet you, virtual-twin.'

Rachel, feeling nauseous, dashed for the sink in the shower room, somehow remembering to shut the door. She was sick immediately, and went on and on, vomiting. Blood kept oozing from her arm. The next thing there was banging in the outer room. Doors banging. Voices raised. She opened the door a crack and then stood there, unsteady.

'The black girl, I said. Rachel. Not *Rachelle*. *Rachel* is the diabetic one. The insulin was for *her*. Didn't you check the name?'

A young doctor was frantically working over the Rachelle girl, struggling to set up a drip. A flurry of nurses salted in and out of the room, arguing. Rachelle, on the bed, looked worse than ever. Scarily still. Withered. Not good. Not good at all.

Rachel, on the step, rocks back and fore, back and fore. She's still rocking, tears flooding her cheeks, when her mother finds her. 'Not your fault.' Her mother tries to take her in her arms. 'You didn't give her the injection.'

'If I'd stayed on my bed … ' Rachel weeps. 'Then I'd have heard. I'd have put them right. Or if I'd not been there at all. Or if I'd taken better care of myself. Or if I'd been at home … '

'Not your fault,' her mother insists. 'No one can say that. Come on – people are staring. You're causing a disturbance.'

Her mother's right. She is. All the folk coming in and out, visitors and staff, are looking at her, staring. Not in a good way. Their eyes seem hard. Rachel feels vulnerable, exposed. It's like they know. It's like she'll never escape this day, this moment. Never.

JAKE: 32 YEARS OLD

The phone rang – although *rang* was not the word, not exactly. The tone was subtle, a mellow sound somehow, as plush as the Chinese rug under his desk. 'Mr Bryan?' His secretary.

'Yes, Amy?'

'It's Mrs Bryan again – your ex-wife, that is: not your mother. It's the third time she's rung.

Oh, and the Jenssens have just been in touch. Delayed. Caught in traffic.'

'Put her through, Amy. Thanks.' Jake sighed. The phone clicked into distant mode. Funny how it did that, gaining an echo, making all voices – Ellie's more than most – unnaturally shrill.

'Jake? Jake? You didn't phone. How did things go?'

'At the hospital?'

'Of course, at the hospital. Where else?' Jake could feel the tension gathering in his spine. Ellie's calls did that to him. When they had been together, she'd driven him up the wall – unremitting, unending interrogation every day. It had been a tirade about his bowels and his skin, masked as sympathetic interest, with Ellie reeling off his litany of defects – the smell in the bathroom, the skin scales on the rug. He struggled for composure, keeping his voice deliberately calm.

'Everything was fine. Doc Martin was pleased.'

'And the blood tests?'

'No problem.'

'And they're continuing the treatment?'

'The NHS is covering patients coming off the trials. For now.'

'And did you ask for a dermatology opinion?'

'On the biologics, my skin's perfect, Ellen.'

Ellen changed tack, abruptly. 'These drugs have side effects, Jake. You want to be careful.' He said nothing. He sighed. Once more, she changed the subject. 'When will you be finished work?' Jake glanced at his diary.

'One more appointment – a civil partnership. I mean, a couple looking for a venue.'

'At the Grosvenor?' Shock sharpened her voice. Ellie could be so *narrow*. How could he ever have interpreted her ignorance as confidence?

'It's just another wedding.'

'If you say so.' She sniffed. 'You promised you'd see Carrie this week.'

'I'll come over soon.' *Carrie was a dog, for heaven's sake. Thank goodness they'd never gone the length of having kids. And thank goodness,* he thought, *for immunosuppressants.* The side effects were rubbish – he'd had plenty of them – but they had won the argument against procreation. Ellie sniffed again.

'I've heard that before.' The phone went dead. Blessed silence.

Jake held the receiver, staring at it. *Why had he married Ellie? What had he seen in her? She'd been his boss's daughter, yes, and Eric had been pleased. But the marriage, from the start, was a disaster.* His skin – so clear in their courtship – relapsed when Eric died. Ellie could not look at him. Flinched when she touched him. Her obsessive interest in his symptoms masked disgust. Disgust and, Jake was sure, disappointment.

Carol, his first girlfriend, had not been like that. Carol was bright. She was lovely. She thought about things – thought them through. Looking at him she had always seen *him*, not the psoriasis. *So why had he ended it? Pushed her away? And Ellie?* he wondered. *Had he done the same with her?*

'Mr Bryan?' Amy popped her head around the door, interrupting his daydreams. 'Your phone's off the hook.'

'Sorry?'

'They're here.' Jake swung around.

'The Jenssens? Bring them up, Amy. Thanks.'

He replaced the receiver, and then he searched in his drawer for the tube of hand cream that Carol had bought him all those years ago. It was still his favourite. Norwegian. That tickled him, somehow. He could not have said why. He worked carefully, efficiently, until every drop of moisture was massaged in, leaving the skin supple, soft. His hands were good now, perfect, but old habits die hard.

LIZ: 40 YEARS OLD

'I'm sorry you missed your last appointment, Mrs Diaz.'

'Miss,' Liz corrected. She nodded. 'Thank you, doctor. I'm sorry, too. I mean, I knew it was around that time, but Sophie had her audition that very day – for the Royal Ballet School. They phoned at the last minute, and it was all such a rush – and they were on the *same* day, you know? And I meant to phone and cancel – thought I had – but obviously – and I didn't remember after that – not until Dr Wocjik got in touch. I am *so* sorry.'

Five years ago. Liz would have died of embarrassment. This time, she got through the interview and examination, if not with actual confidence, with less anxiety. She had become used to the routine check-ups, to the examination, to the period of waiting for results, if it was always too long.

The doctor was still talking as Liz reached the door. 'And you'll need six-monthly smears, of course.'

'Smears?'

'Your GP will do them for you.'

'But you do them here … ' The doctor looked confused.

'Mrs – Miss – Diaz, I've just been explaining that we can discharge you now, back to your own doctor's care.'

'Discharge?'

'Discharge.'

'You mean everything's fine?'

'Yes.' The doctor sighed. 'Absolutely fine, Mrs – Ms Diaz. We can leave things in your own doctor's hands. Dr Wocjik will look after you from now on. You're happy with that?'

'Wonderfully.' Liz beamed. 'That's absolutely marvellous. Thank you, Doctor Gupta.'

She hesitated, blushing, her hand on the door knob.

'Yes? You have a question?'

'If – if I was considering a future pregnancy?'

'Well … ' The doctor nodded. 'Perhaps we should discuss this. Come back. Sit down.' Liz remained standing by the door.

Dr Gupta referred to her notes. 'Let me see … you had the first LLETZ carried out five years ago for CIN2. Then, two years ago, you had another episode of dyskariotic change noted. This time CIN1 also treated with LLETZ, which has – so far at least – remained clear. It is harder, of course, to assess these things in pregnancy.' She looked up. 'And 36 years is not altogether young for a pregnancy. Fertility is not as buoyant either – not as reliable. There's a small risk of low birthweight and early delivery even with the LLETZ. And other risks as well. Down's syndrome increases with maternal age, as will the risk of twins, but you will know these things, I'm sure. You will have read them on the Internet. You are hoping for another pregnancy? It is on the cards?'

Liz's blush deepened. 'I'm not sure. I wondered about my medication.'

'Medication?' Dr Gupta flicked back through the notes. 'Ah. For epilepsy? You are still being treated for that?' Liz nodded. 'But you had no problems last time. Has your prescription changed?'

'I still take Valproate, but the dose is lower.'

'And do you still have fits?'

'Not for the last two years.'

'Then it may be safer to try stopping the treatment altogether. Or perhaps to modify the way you take the drug. Also you would need folic acid, which can protect against foetal abnormality. You will remember from last time that even epilepsy itself can be associated with a small increase in risk for the child? But it would be best to discuss all this at length.' Dr Gupta looked at the clock and sighed. It's not absolutely straightforward. I'll tell you what, Mrs Diaz, would you like me to book you into our pre-conception clinic? It would be for the best. You must take time over this. ' Liz nodded.

'But Sophie was perfect.'

'Shall I book you in? You must bring your partner along. We'll discuss everything – all the aspects, and help you come to a decision. Come, sit down. Let me find you an appointment.'

'Thank you.' Liz remained where she was. 'Perhaps you would send it out?'

Dr Gupta reeled through a set of options on the computer screen and tapped her mouse twice. 'There. You can collect the card on your way out. Appointment in two months. Ask at the desk. You are using contraception?'

'I'm still on the pill. Dr Wocjik thought that was the safest option.'

'Then please continue that for the moment. And make no change to your other medication until you come to the pre-conception clinic. You must have the best of information before you make this important decision. I wish we had the time today … ' She shook her head. 'But you can see how busy the waiting room is.'

'Thank you, doctor. Thank you for your time.'

As Liz made her escape, Dr Gupta spoke again. 'And what about your daughter?'

'My daughter?'

'Yes. How did the audition go?'

'We haven't heard yet,' Liz responded. 'We're still hoping.'

'You must be very proud of her.'

'Oh yes, Dr Gupta.' Liz smiled. 'We all are. Very proud indeed.'

JEN AND GEOFF

Five years to the day, Jane returned to the cemetery armed with freesias – red and yellow – and maidenhair fern. Jen's favourites. The graveyard, as always, was oddly cheering. Birds whistled in the branches of the tall beech trees beyond the canal. Jen would have liked that. She loved to watch the birds.

It broke Jane's heart reading through the calendar her sister had kept on her kitchen wall.

Siskins today. Saw the wren! Visited Geoff.

Hospice today. Dr Friend. Told him about the woodpecker.

First martins this year.

'No siskins here, Jen. But you'd like that blackbird's song.' Jane poured water into the vase set before the gravestone. *In loving memory*, it said. *Dearly beloved wife and mother. Much loved sister.* Jane shook her head. 'Saw Geoff this morning,' she chatted, ripping the cellophane from the flowers. 'He looks very comfortable. Doesn't get around much, but they had him sitting up, watching TV, when I went in.'

This was not a lie. The TV had been on, and Geoff sitting, staring at it, blank as the white wall behind him. Like he always had been. Jane shook her head and tried to think better of the man. After all, her twin had loved him. It would have hurt her to the bone to see him propped there like that, leaning to one side. Utterly vacant. He'd collapsed into himself once Jen had gone, as if her love, her will, had been the last thing pinning him to reality.

Sometimes, he'd been angry, even violent, when Jane had come to visit. Once, he had tried to hit her. At least he was quiet now. *Was he sedated?* Jane never asked. And they were good in the home; they talked to him all the time, as if he had a chance of understanding. They were much more patient than she would have been. It was hard enough to just sit there for half an hour.

Geoff had his own room at the back of the building – a comfortable room, very fresh. It never smelled of urine. Or soup. That was something Jen had always hated – the reek of stale soup. Nurses were in and out all the time, checking and fixing Geoff. They'd even brought her tea. Told her he was eating better. 'Has his daughter been in?' The Matron shook her head. 'Likely, she finds it hard, after all the legal hassle,' said Jane. 'Difficult for her to accept that everything was in Jen's name, willed to me after she was gone. The boy understood, but of course he's in the States … I don't suppose he's in touch either?'

'Not in the last year, no.'

'Well, the legal challenge is sorted at last, and the house sold. Everything's gone through. Not that the sale did more than cover legal costs. And the remortgage, of course. That wasn't a bad thing – made their last years together more comfortable than they may have been. When I was clearing the house I found these things and I've brought them for him.'

'Where would you like me to leave them?'

She'd spread out the wedding photographs, his precious gardening books, and all the photographs of the garden, too. She had left them on the table beside the television but Geoff had paid them no notice, or at least none that she could see.

'So, Jen,' she finished briskly. 'he looked very well. I'll look in on him again when I come back. On your birthday.' She pulled herself to her feet. 'I'll not be back before then, but I phone the home every week, like I promised. He's very peaceful, lass. Looks well. I think he's put on a bit of weight.'

Not until she'd reached the cemetery gate did she realise that she'd not told her twin the most important thing of all. 'As if you'd hear it any better over there!' All the same, she turned towards the grave, visualising Jen as she'd been when they were 30 – not the worn-out scrap of life, the skin and bones and burning eyes she'd nursed through the agony and grief of those last long days.

Not the poor, aching mite who could bear the pain of turning in the bed but not the fear of what may befall Geoff when she was gone. Jane banished such images. Nor did she picture her sister at the end in that bleak hospital bed – unconscious, wracked in a desperate symphony of rasping, failing breath.

Whoever said it was easy to die in bed? They knew nothing about it. Nothing.

These Jens had existed, but they were not *Jen*. They did not define her and Jane spoke to her sister at 30 – no, *29:* the day before Jen met and was beguiled by Geoff – the last day she and Jen had been truly inseparable.

'What I meant to tell you is that Jack's Courtney – his youngest – had her baby last week, at last. And you'll never guess? They've only gone and called her Jennifer-Jane! Both our names – one child! What d' you think of that? She looks exactly like us. You're a great-grand-aunt, Jen! And I'm a great grandmother, although I haven't seen the baby – haven't had a cuddle – just a photo. Bye, then, lass. I'll have to go; I can see the bus coming up the hill. Not so quick on my pins these days.'

She walked towards the bus stop, facing resolutely forward. These trips were important but exhausting. All she had to do now was to reach the station and the waiting train. She'd be home by nine.

What's it all about? she wondered, not for the first time. *Life. Where does it take us? What does it all mean? What is it for? Look at us. Poor Jen gone. Geoff a vegetable. Not that I ever liked the man. The baby, though. The baby is a good thing. A baby with both our names. Jen would have loved that.*

2

A piece of my skin: a physician facing his future

RAIMO PUUSTINEN

I

I am a doctor. That means that I should know. And I do know.

When I first noticed that change on my forehead, I knew that men over 50 have certain kinds of changes in their skin because of their age. That particular change of my skin was small, round and smooth and it did not bother me a bit. But then my wife told me that it makes me look like an old man, because old men have all kinds of spots on their foreheads, and she does not want to be married to an old man as yet (although she also is over 50 and she has those small brownish spots on her skin). I told her that I'll get rid of my spot as soon as I find time to have it removed.

I did not find the time to have it removed. Then the lesion started to change. Now, since I am a doctor, I knew that it was no longer merely a cosmetic issue, but there obviously was something going on in my skin that should not be going on there. The smooth surface on the lesion got bumpy and the skin started to peel off, with some slight itching. I decided that it looked pretty much like a basal cell carcinoma (BCC), a type of a skin cancer. As a physician I knew that it is a 'benign' condition in the sense that it will not kill me. I also knew that I had better have it removed while it was small, that is, while it has not grown all over my face. The theoretical problem was, however, that I was a bit young (objectively speaking) to develop a basal cell carcinoma and that my lesion had grown quite rapidly, in a matter of weeks, which is somewhat atypical for BCCs.

So, to please my wife and to live up to my professional standards, I called a friend of mine, a plastic surgeon, to take a look at my forehead. He scrutinised my skin in his nicely decorated surgery, using the latest imaging technology that he has purchased to deal with his mainly wealthy female patients. He photographed my spot, downloaded the picture to his Mac and magnified it on the screen. We took a good look at it and agreed that it looked pretty much like a basal cell carcinoma. We decided that we had better have it removed before it has the chance to grow any bigger.

I soon found myself lying on his operating table. My lesion had grown to the size of an almond and he had to remove quite a bit of my forehead to get the whole thing off. He dropped that piece of my skin into a small bottle filled with formalin and stitched my head with all of his plastic surgeon's skills. When he finished he told me that he would send that piece of my skin to a pathologist for further evaluation. The nurse advised me to have the stitches removed after 10–14 days and gave me a leaflet with detailed instructions of how to deal with the wound. And that was that.

So, I kept on living and working as usual and my staff and patients were courteous enough not to make any queries about the band aid and stitches on my forehead. I just kept changing the dressings and had the stitches removed as planned. The wound was healing *per primam intentionem*, as we doctors like to say.

Then my colleague called me. He said he had received the pathologist's report. It was not a basal cell carcinoma. The moment I heard my colleague's voice I knew there was something seriously wrong with my skin; and not just my skin, but my whole body and eventually my whole existence. I kept my professional attitude and did not allow myself to sink into existential agonies, but concentrated on the facts.

The facts were that in that piece of my skin was a pile of nasty-looking lymphocytes that should not have been there, or anywhere else for that matter, meaning that I most likely had a lymphoma, another form of a cancer.

II

My friend then told me that that little piece of my skin had been sent to the local university hospital for further evaluation and that I should be contacted by them soon. He said he was sorry. I knew he was. After all, he was my friend and a doctor. And as doctors we know only too well that when things start to go wrong they can go seriously wrong. And of all people, we know what can and what cannot be done to get them right again.

So I did what every seasoned doctor would do. I consulted Google. After all, how often does an ordinary GP have to deal with T- or B- or whatever-cell lymphomas? Practically never. Lymphomas are dealt with by those who end up working at the university hospital. If I should ever diagnose a syllable-something-lymphoma in any of my patients I would refer them to someone whose job it is to deal with such biological oddities. As a GP I just need to recognise those oddities from among an endless stream of aches, pains, fears and worries and all the other problems my patients present to me every day.

But now it was the question of *my* skin, and as a physician I knew that I was facing a potentially lethal problem. So, I did the next thing that every sensible doctor would do in those circumstances; I consulted a lawyer, to ensure that I would not leave my family with the outrageous mortgage, based on my illusion of being immortal and making a decent living from doctoring forever.

While I knew that the skin lesion on my forehead was removed for good, I had no idea whether there was more of that malignant tissue on the loose, rampaging through my body. I was about to find out. I was invited to the university hospital to have my whole body scanned, while the pathologists were figuring out how to categorise the anomalous piece of skin tissue.

I had never been in that huge complex as a patient, the very complex where I had received my medical training decades ago. Now the complex was much, much bigger than in those days.

I did manage to find my way to the dermatology outpatient clinic, following the signs and asking the cleaning lady to be sure. After browsing some yester-year magazines, I was invited into a nice, clean and wholly impersonal room to see a dermatologist. She was, I was assured by my plastic surgeon friend, the number one lymphoma specialist in this part of the country.

The doctor knew that I was a physician, too, and that I, therefore, knew the facts. She said that the piece of skin had already been evaluated by three pathologists, and that the one to give the final verdict is the number one expert in the whole country. That is one of the benefits of being a physician: you get the best there is just by being a member of the fraternity.

The problem with that piece of my skin, however, was that its cellular structure did not seem to fit any of the prevailing categories in the way we classify lymphomas today. The conclusion was that, for the time being, it might just be a benign phenomenon after all. Perhaps there was nothing to worry about, but further tests were needed, just to be sure.

Nothing to worry about? Gosh. My wife had gone to pieces when I had told her about the initial pathologist's report. Well, actually, I did not tell her. She happened to notice the letter from the clinic, and she forced me to tell her what it was all about. Meanwhile, I had visited London for my pre-planned trip to examine old medical textbooks at the Wellcome Library, so that I could write an essay on prognosis for this book. What a trip. There I was sitting in the library, knowing that I had a lymphoma, browsing through dusty books and planning my funeral.

And now I was in that sterile, well-lit examination room at the university hospital and the dermatologist was telling me that the lesion could just be a haphazard phenomenon and that it had been completely removed by the plastic surgeon friend of mine; but …

The word But is a very important word in medicine. In fact, medicine is built on Buts. I use it all the time with my patients. 'You have this-and-this, take that-and-that and you'll be well in so-and-so-many-days or so-and-so-many-weeks; *but* if you are not, call me.'

So, the dermatologist said that there was nothing to worry about. But, just to make sure, it would be good to run some further tests. Further tests? Why? Didn't she just say there was nothing to worry about? This all started to sound like a very interesting epistemological problem.

III

I then found myself sitting at 7.50 on another Monday morning at a University Hospital Radiology Department with a couple of other terrified-looking people, watching the early morning television show and pretending that we are not there for any serious reason.

Came then a male nurse with a tray full of jars filled with opaque liquid. He placed three of these in front of each of us and said we should drink the stuff over the next two hours. The truck-driver-looking guy next to me sighed and said there was a lot to drink. I comforted him by suggesting that we should pretend that they are three pints, which was not much to consume in two hours in a pub. We toast and start the slow drinking.

After I had filled my guts with that dull-tasting stuff I was invited into the X-ray computed tomography (CT)-scan room. A blonde nurse gave me the details of what was going to happen in the next ten minutes or so. I had to change my clothes for a gown and she installed a catheter in my left arm. She told me that l will be injected with some material that will help to recognise different tissues in my body in the pictures to come. I didn't tell her that I knew all that.

She departed and I was laying still. I heard a humming sound and saw whirling lights moving across my body. I heard the nurse's voice from the loudspeaker: 'Inhale. Hold your breath. Breathe.' I did as I was told. I heard her voice again: 'You will feel a warm sensation descending from your head to your legs while we are injecting the liquid into your veins.' And, indeed, after a while I did feel this odd sensation of heat going through my body, descending to my groins as if I had wet my pants. I felt a short spell of nausea and then it was all over. The nurse appeared by my side, took out the needle and told me to dress and go back to the information desk to get my number for the next procedure.

I felt dizzy putting my shirt on. I imagined my colleagues sitting in a darkened room and examining the shades of grey on their screens, representing the order of my tissues, and discerning whether there is something that should not be there.

I left the examining room and grinned at those sitting looking nervous and pretending they are not. I felt like telling the truck-driver-looking guy that it will not be all that bad, that the nurse is good looking, that it didn't hurt and so on, but I said nothing. I just went to the office as instructed to provide information as instructed for what the dermatologist had entered into the hospital computer.

The lady at the desk gave me a number and directed me to another waiting lounge, saying that I would be called for further procedures in due course. I sat for a while and then another blonde nurse called me in. She was one of those no-nonsense types, telling me to take my shirt off and lie on the examination table. I did what she said and she left the room, dimming the lights on her way out.

I lay on the couch and wait for what seemed to be a long time. Just before reaching my irritation level a young female physician arrived. She introduced herself and I muttered something in reply. She looked at my chart on the screen and recognised my profession. A colleague, she noted. I said 'No, I am a patient.' She smiled and got into her ultrasound business. I got a lot of that cold and slimy stuff around my neck and she started probing my body with her scanners.

She was very matter of fact, but somehow I felt the tension in her, probably because I was a colleague and brought into relief the vulnerability of our bodies. Being a doctor does not protect us, even though we like to think that somehow it does. I felt the probe going up and down my neck. Routine. Good news. Stopping and going the same route again, and again. Bad news. As a doctor I knew what was going on. She had spotted something that shouldn't be there. Finally, she told the nurse to prepare for a biopsy. She then explained to me that she needed to take a specimen of tissue, just to make sure. I heard that she was trying to sound as if there was nothing to worry about. But I knew that there was.

The nurse prepared the equipment and washed my neck. It was kind of amusing to see how these people were more conscientious with all the hygiene control than I was in my own surgery. But I did not mind; I'd rather not have any of the germs they host in their thoroughly clean premises.

When the nurse was ready, the physician stuck a needle into my right parotid area. That hurt. She started to hoover my cells into a syringe. When she was satisfied she pulled the needle out and asked whether I was going to see any patients that day. I told her that no, I was not. I had expected that I would be more or less sick with all the stuff injected into me and sucked out of me and that I most likely would not have been in the mood to see any patients with their ordinary aches, pains, worries and sorrows. None of that for that day. I had plenty of my own worry.

I got back to my business-as-usual life and waited for the results. It took a fortnight for the dermatologist to get all the material together and make up her mind what that cluster of anomalous cells was all about. She called me while I was examining a patient. I told my patient that there was a hospital doctor consulting me and I left the room with my cell phone to hear and face the facts as a physician. The dermatologist congratulated me and said that the number one pathologist in the country had decided that my lesion was a benign, but rather rare, phenomenon and my body scan, ultrasound sample and the gallon of blood, urine and tissue samples I had given for laboratory tests were all normal. But, she said, if anything suspicious should appear in the future I should not hesitate to call her any time.

I went back to my office to continue with the bad hip and felt a bit lighter. Quite a bit, I must say. I felt like I had somehow got my life back, even though I had just been concentrating on the facts throughout the whole process. You see, I am a doctor. I concentrate on facts. I know how things are, and how they are going to be.

Giving a prognosis is not difficult. I know that one day my body will break down and I will die. I also know that I don't know how and when that will happen. In fact, it is quite comforting to know that one does not know – one of the privileges of being a doctor.

3

Prognosis as process

ROLF AHLZÉN

Patients, as their illness has been given a name, usually ask next: And how long will it take? How long will it be before …? How long? How long? And the doctor replies that he cannot promise but … He can appear to be the controller of time, as, on occasions, the mariner appears to rule the sea. But both mariner and doctor know this to be an illusion.[1]

INTRODUCTION

A peculiar ambiguity is associated with the notion of prognosis. Prognosis is often thought of as a physician's prediction about the probable development and outcome of a disease. It may, however, also refer to the actual course of the disease. The former may be distinguished as prognostication, while the latter can be seen as prognosis proper. Prognosis may also refer to an ill person's reflections on what will happen now and in the distant future. The illness experience may be filled with hope and despair, fear and trust. 'What will this disease do to me?' The crucial importance of the patient's anticipation of the future, the *prognosis-as-lived*, is easily overlooked.

A common cold means quick recovery, while a cancer diagnosis carries the weight of possible decay and death. Some diagnoses are trivial; some are dreaded. What diseases actually do to us is the core of both diagnosis and prognosis. Prognosis can therefore be seen as the affective side of diagnosis, as diagnosis coloured by prognosis.

My intention is an exploration of the interrelationship between these three aspects of prognosis, and how these develop over time. Physicians are expected to prognosticate, while ill people inevitably experience distress, or even anguish, facing an uncertain future. The disease runs its biological course, more or less affected by medical interventions, but we need to look closely at how the medically defined disease, the pathological process in the body, interacts with the lived experience of being ill.

As John Berger notes, uncertainty permeates both prognostication and the illness experience. But while uncertainty for the ill person may shake the very foundations of existence, the difficulty of medical prediction is largely due to the complexities of biological processes, and, as we shall see, the physician's own fears about how he or she thinks the patient may respond.

SHOULD PHYSICIANS PROGNOSTICATE?

Rachel, in our stories, is diagnosed with diabetes; Liz has an atypical cervical smear; Jake has an irritable bowel and psoriasis. Do we find their doctors telling them that their diagnoses will probably mean this or that for their lives in the future? Do they give them a good idea about what they may expect? Do they talk to them about what is known and not known about the future course of their diseases? In fact we read very little about these aspects of the consultations. Physician and sociologist Nicholas Christakis would see this as a confirmation of his thesis that physicians fail in their responsibility to prognosticate, as well as to take an active interest in their patients' thoughts, fears and hopes for the future. In *Death Foretold: prophecy and prognosis in medical care*, he argues that 'compassionate responses' to patients' requests for prognosis are an essential part of the physician's task and that doctors far too often abdicate this responsibility.[2]

Prognostication, notes Christakis, is used not only for the purpose of illuminating therapeutic options it also is 'used by physicians, both advertently and inadvertently, to fulfil other objectives such as fostering compliance, cultivating hope, managing expectations, relieving anxiety, and engendering confidence'.[3] It is worth adding that the relative importance of these other uses of prognosis changes over time. While it may be advisable for Rachel's physician, immediately after a diagnosis of diabetes, to give her a prognosis that emphasises hope, it may be just as important to warn about the long-term complications at a later stage, should Rachel's resistance to therapy endanger her future health.

The obvious reason why physicians should prognosticate is that most ill people want them to. At an early stage, while there may still be diagnostic uncertainty, the wise physician is often very cautious. When investigating a person for a potentially grave symptom, where a cancer is possible but unlikely, it may actually be unethical to present a series of stark prognoses. However, if a cancer diagnosis is confirmed, it will be of the utmost importance for the patient to hear his or her physician inform him or her about the prospects for the future. These will include therapeutic options, effects and side effects of treatment, chances for remission, risks of relapse and long-term survival. Christakis presents ample empirical evidence that doctors often fail in these responsibilities.

Uncertainty may be one reason for doctors to hesitate when their patients ask them about their future, but a prognosis that emphasises uncertainty is still a prognosis. For several chronic diseases of autoimmune origin, prognosis at an early stage is exceedingly difficult, due both to diagnostic uncertainty and the wide range of possible courses that the disease may take. A rheumatoid arthritis that initially seems calm and slowly progressing may suddenly change character and become more aggressive. Ulcerative colitis may have an acute onset, but when properly treated remain silent for a long time. To prognosticate about the frequency and severity of relapses is impossible. But this knowledge is also a prognosis, albeit one that stresses uncertainty.

Physicians may also avoid prognosticating for fear of their patients' reactions. More or less consciously they may assume that a gloomy prognosis works as a self-fulfilling prophecy and that inducing hopelessness may facilitate progression or recurrence of disease. Hope, it is then assumed, works therapeutically. Christakis notes:

> Overall, physicians correct patient pessimism and reinforce patient optimism. These behaviour patterns manifested themselves even when the patient was quite sick.[4]

A physician reacting to an illness with a prognosis emphasising optimism against the odds, may inadvertently make it more difficult for the patient to cope with whatever comes. Premature reassurance may be counterproductive and pave the way for disappointment and distrust, failure to follow recommendations or unrealistic plans for the future.

A common source of uncertainty in prognostication is patients' very different responses to treatment. Often, physicians hesitate to say much about their patients' prospects before they have seen how they react to therapy. The patient's response to treatment may change the prognosis; a good response to treatment may mean that the overall prognosis is greatly improved. Hence, prognostication is subject to constant evaluation and re-evaluation.

Patients may reject prognostication. They may want to know only parts of what the physician finds out about their diseases. They may even reject all information about tests and treatments. In the extreme case, fear of the prognosis may lead patients to avoid finding out about their diagnosis altogether. In Lars Gustafsson's novel *The Death of a Beekeeper*, the main character, who has for a time suffered from increasingly severe pain in his upper abdomen, burns the brown envelope from the hospital that he is certain will give him the truth. His repression of diagnosis comes with his fear of lethal prognosis.[5]

PROGNOSIS-AS-LIVED

Prognostication deals with disease as a biological phenomenon, attempting to predict how pathological processes in the body will develop over time. Prognosis-as-lived is about illness, the uniquely individual anticipation of the way that a disease influences and changes one's future. Both change due to the ongoing processes in the body, but also due to the interplay between these bodily changes and the ill person's interpretations – and due to the relation between the ill person and others, among whom physicians hold a key position. The course of the disease is intimately connected to the physician's prognostication because it is governing what is said to the patient and which measures are deemed meaningful. The course of the disease is also affected by the patient's lifestyle and compliance with treatment – these too are aspects of the prognosis-as-lived.

Diagnosis is permeated by the future. It points to options lost, dreams obstructed and challenges to be faced. For the ill person, every diagnostic label carries implications for the weeks, months or years to come. These may be vague and largely unknown, as in a disease like systemic lupus erythematosis (SLE), which has unpredictable effects on different organ systems at highly irregular intervals and seldom any identifiable precipitating factors. Or they may be well defined and controllable, like a gastric ulcer due to an infection with helicobacter pylori, which can be eradicated with a low risk of recurrence. It is not difficult to see how such conditions pose different challenges to the ill person.

Individual reactions to diagnosis are strikingly different. Fears may be exaggerated in contrast to biomedical facts. Wishful thinking may, on the contrary, lead to repression of a dismal prognosis. It is the prognostic implications of diagnosis that make individual reactions to them vary so immensely, in combination with individual variability in reaction to threats and challenges. As mentioned, Lars Gustafsson's beekeeper rejects diagnosis for fear of prognosis. This remains the central enigma of the novel. In our stories, when Liz received information about the cervical smear, she was not able to handle it rationally, and she did not get the right help to do so. It is only now, when we meet her again, sometime later, that she has come to terms with her situation and is looking to the future. Insensitivity on the side of the physician increased her fear. Rachel, on the other hand, was fortunate to get the support she needed to help her to understand and handle her diabetes. Her fears are probably not due to lack of information or professional insensitivity but rather to the predicament of being a teenager who cannot be expected to handle long-term complex projections very rationally. The physician and other professionals like the diabetes nurse can contribute to a balanced interpretation of the consequences of diagnosis, but patients' secret fears can remain hidden, even from the most insightful helper. In our story, Rachel sees herself as responsible for the harm coming to another young woman who receives her dose of insulin by mistake. How will this affect the lived prognosis for her?

A disease that is labelled 'minor' may have symptoms that are not very problematic to handle and that are over in a short time. A urinary infection is an obvious example. However, if the infection is the seventh in as many months, it will carry a totally different meaning, and its prognosis may take on a grave importance. 'Will this ever end?' is the natural question that the physician is expected to answer. So it is that diagnoses receive their emotional colouring from their prognoses.

At first the patient's imagining of his or her future situation is influenced by a number of diagnostic possibilities from the trivial to the very serious. The ill person may be thrown between hope and despair. With a disease like cancer of the colon the prognosis largely depends on the existence of distant metastases. The results of a single ultrasound of the liver may mean the difference between many more years of life or a very gloomy prognosis. With every new step in the diagnostic process, more information is gained and prognostication usually becomes easier. For the patient, this means relief or anguish, hope or despair.

Symptoms may be interpreted as dangerous even without a medical diagnosis. A middle-aged man once told me that when his first child was born, he became intensely worried that he had a serious disease. For three weeks he was extremely tense, fearing that he would not be given the chance to see his newly born daughter grow up. When he met his physician on the day of the gastroscopy, he told him about his anxiety, which he thought was both embarrassing and inexplicable. The physician calmly looked at him and uttered: 'It is not at all hard to understand, when you realise what is at stake.' These few words had a strongly consoling effect on him. He came to see them not only as well chosen for the moment, but as carrying a deeper truth about his existential predicament. He was found to be fully healthy.

Screening procedures for diseases such as breast cancer (mammography), cervical cancer (smears) and prostate cancer (PSA-tests) may be followed by delays, characteristic of many healthcare systems, leaving patients in a state of unnecessary anxiety. The very existence of these procedures may induce a chronic uncertainty about people's health, even when they feel healthy. The taken-for-granted trust in the future, at least the near future, which follows from experiencing health, is undermined. Prognosis-as-lived is shaken by the constant reminder of hidden dangers, silent bodily processes gone wrong.

LIVED EXPERIENCE AND BIOLOGICAL PROCESSES

How does prognosis-as-lived affect the course of a disease and the prognosis? We do not know whether thoughts, feelings, expectations and assumptions have psychophysical correlates that influence pathophysiological processes. Recommendations for 'positive thinking' were fashionable some years ago. There was little evidence to support this, partly because the whole notion of 'positive thinking' remained obscure. It is now clear that such effects, if they exist at all, are of limited importance compared with other factors influencing the course of a disease. A well-founded ethical objection to these ideas proposed that they merely induced guilt in people who were not capable of such thinking.

It seems clear, however, that the lived prognosis influences the ill person's self-understanding, which in turn affects the way he or she complies with treatments as well as the structure of his or her everyday life – eating, drinking, exercise, sleep and so forth. These are factors that govern the patient's ability to 'run the race' imposed by a disease. Pessimism and passivity arising from a harsh prognosis may be followed by behaviours that often decrease the body's capacity to regain balance and face painful or demanding treatments.

The onset of somatic disease may be followed by disappointment and anger over lost possibilities. These may, step by step, deepen into a mental state where all hope is gone and only darkness and meaninglessness remain. Depression is lived prognosis turned into merciless darkness. For the ill person, it is the end of prognosis. For the physician, depression creates a new challenge to add to the challenge of managing the somatic disease. Depression secondary to grave disease means much suffering for the ill person, and dramatically changes the prognosis for the worse – at least if it is not properly and urgently treated. The ultimate and deeply tragic consequence of an untreated depression may be suicide.

A particular emotional challenge is offered by chronic diseases that run with long free intervals and occasional relapses. In SLE, an autoimmune disease of connective tissues, relapses are feared because they are often followed by further loss of function. Medication or other interventions to reduce the risk of relapse may induce difficult side effects. Several of the drugs used for the treatment of chronic psychiatric disorders, like bipolar disorder or schizophrenia, cause serious side effects, necessitating difficult negotiations within the ill person and with the physician.

FROM POPULATION TO INDIVIDUAL

Prognostication is largely based on generalisation from population studies. It is the clinician's task to try to translate this into a prognosis for each unique case, and to help the ill person to accept and live with the inevitable uncertainty involved. The physician's expertise concerns the medical prognosis but, as this aspect of prognosis is deeply intertwined with the lived prognosis, the good physician cannot avoid the patient's subjective experience.

The 'treatment' of risk factors offers particular challenges. Increasing segments of the population are taking preventive measures for marginal gains. These interventions are based on data from large epidemiological studies on selected populations, statistically linking certain biomedical parameters – like blood pressure, lipid levels or blood glucose – to the incidence of certain diseases over a period of time. In manipulating these parameters, physicians try to slow the course of an initially asymptomatic bodily process, such as atherosclerosis. This is treatment exclusively for changing a statistically defined group prognosis, which may or may not affect any one of the people in the group.

There are considerable difficulties here. Medication often carries the risk of side effects. Prognostication from populations to individuals is fundamentally uncertain and theoretical risk reduction may be actual or illusory. Side effects of interventions are difficult to foresee. Some patients may suffer seriously reduced quality of life without their prognosis (to stay healthy or avoid relapse) being improved at all. For others it may be the other way around. Risks are, by definition, experienced by different individuals in a non-foreseeable manner.

Feeling well and being declared at risk means being told that my well-being is an illusion and that threatening things are going on silently and invisibly in my body. My way of looking at my future may be transformed, slightly or considerably. Biomedical prognosis acts imperialistically in relation to my lived experience. This is medicalisation in its very essence – benevolent, at times successful as a preventive tool, but also carrying obvious risks of undermining our reliance on our bodies and our trust in the future. Benevolent intentions may here prove counter-productive in a broader perspective.

A study by Swedish anthropologist Lisbeth Sachs showed that a group of elderly men, diagnosed with high levels of blood lipids, were told that it would be good to change diet and medicate with statins, due to 'long term' risks of complications. When interviewed about their interpretations of this, it was found that a majority handled the information in a sensible way, realising that this was not much to worry about, just an ordinary precautionary measure to avoid problems in the future. A considerable number, however, went home and started to imagine small white projectiles that would at any moment obstruct a vessel in the heart or brain. Their lives were radically changed and their earlier trust in their bodily being was replaced by a fundamental existential uncertainty.[6]

Even with a reasonably good medical prognosis, the lived prognosis may be difficult to handle. A statistically good prognosis in relation to a fatal outcome (like a 93% five-year survival in a malignant disease) still means an estimated 7% risk to die in five years. How can such a statistically based answer to the patient's question about the prognosis possibly be transformed into real lived experience? Who can handle this 7% figure in a rational way? What does 'rational' mean in the context of life and death? The physician may attempt to translate this 93% into phrases like, 'You stand a very good chance of surviving this cancer,' or 'The odds are very good that the cancer will not come back.' Many ill people will be satisfied with this, but some will ask for more precision: 'Give me the numbers!' or, 'I want to know the risk that I will die, not the chance that I will survive!'

PLACEBO AS PROGNOSIS

What is usually called the placebo effect is the influence on the prognosis of certain contextual factors around investigation, diagnosis and therapy. These may involve the ill person's presuppositions about the disorder and its treatment, as well as the capacity of the physician (or another professional) to induce trust and hope. Puustinen and Louhiala reject the placebo concept as a way of capturing this, as it is so closely associated to the use of 'placebo pills' in randomised controlled trials. They suggest the 'care effect' as a better alternative. The care effect is 'the consequence of the experience of being cared for'.[7] Moerman uses the concept 'meaning effect'.[8] Common to both is the positive effect on prognosis that results from hope and trust.

In relation to the concept of prognosis, the care effect may be seen as the influence that the perceived prognosis has on both the biologically defined disease and on illness, prognosis-as-lived. It is interesting to attempt to distinguish between the two. If the ill person deeply trusts the physician's ability to cure, he or she may be more likely to respond to therapy. But what does it mean to respond? Obviously, the lived prognosis has been influenced, evidenced by the fact that the person feels better and believes that the disease process is being overcome, but what about the actual biological course of the disease? And what of the situation, as outlined by Jill Gordon in Chapter 7, in which 'care' is in fact exploitation for financial gain?

Kaptchuk *et al.* have, in a series of elegant experiments, shown that sham acupuncture has a substantial effect on patients' subjective experiences of asthma. Patients report increased well-being; they think that their disease has lost some of its strength. However, these perceptions are not reflected in an increase in lung capacity, measured as the forced expiratory volume. (FEV).[9] The lung capacity is the same as it was before treatment. It seems that the placebo, or the care effect, has had an effect on the lived prognosis but not on the medical prognosis, at least not in the short run. Is this benefit not good enough, one may ask? What a person thinks and feels surely matters. One may of course argue that this placebo-induced amelioration could cause harm by inducing a patient to withdraw from effective therapy, but this seems unlikely.

Prognosis-as-lived is thus closely linked to caring for, giving hope. Is this the reason why physicians, as Christakis notes, exaggerate optimistic aspects of prognosis for their patients? Is this a rational hope for better life-quality, the opposite of the fear of dire self-fulfilling prophecies? But if an overly optimistic prognosis lets patients down, and they inevitably realise their true prognosis – then this is the opposite of caring. The care effect will, ideally, work for reasons other than unwarranted optimism. Physicians who do not desert their patients, who stand by their side and who give them help and support, fully employ placebo healing.

PAST AND FUTURE

Human beings are by necessity oriented both to the past and the future. We live in a stream of time, as Carl Edvard Rudebeck explores in the chapter that follows. Disease interrupts this flow and demands reorientation, new meaning patterns and reconsideration of central values – both of the past and the future. The time horizon may radically change. Living two more months may mean seeing the birth of a grandchild or experiencing one more spring – the song of birds and green leaves on the trees. There may be deep gratitude for each new day that had earlier been taken for granted. Prognostication forms the lived prognosis, the ill person's hope or fear for the coming months and years. Sensibly and sensitively handled, it opens up consolation and reconciliation. As such it may be, at one and the same time, the most difficult and the noblest of the physician's tasks.

REFERENCES

1. Berger J, Mohr J. *A Fortunate Man: the story of a country doctor.* Vintage; 1997.
2. Christakis NA. *Death Foretold: prophecy and prognosis in medical care.* Chicago, CA: University of Chicago Press; 1999.
3. Ibid. p. 27.
4. Ibid. p. 128.
5. Gustafsson L. *The Death Of a Beekeeper.* New York, NY: New Directions; 1981.
6. Sachs L. Patologi eller ej, det –r frågan? Om de sjuka i v–lf–rdssamh–llet. In: Lagercrantz R, editor. *Andens kraft.* Stockholm: Socialdepartementet; 1996. pp. 63–87.
7. Louhiala P, Puustinen R. Rethinking the placebo effect. *Medical Humanities,* 2008; **34**: 107–9.
8. Moerman, DE. Meaningful placebos – controlling the uncontrollable. *N Engl J Med.* 2011; **365**(2): 171–2.
9. Wechsler ME, Kelley JM, Boyd IO, *et al.* Active albuterol or placebo, sham acupuncture, or no intervention in asthma. *N Engl J Med.* 2011; **365**(2): 119–26.

4

Prognosis, time and commitment

CARL EDVARD RUDEBECK

TIME

In this chapter I will use the freedom invited by writing to focus on time as a decisive element of prognosis, and in fact as an essential element of the doctor–patient relationship itself. As we have seen in these stories, when the doctor senses the future of, not only the disease, but of the patient having the disease, prognostic judgement and care become inseparable. This relation between time and moral commitment is the theme of this chapter. To try to bring the reader on track, we need to begin with some points on the subject of time itself. This should make it easier to see how and when the future becomes the main issue of the present of consultations. We will also see more clearly the distinction between prognosis as science-based and probabilistic reasoning and prognosis as a disclosure of time that morally frames the doctor–patient relationship. In the latter part of the chapter I deal more extensively with the stories of Anne Macleod, as they develop through the whole series of four books. It has given me the opportunity to apply the idea of 'personal prognosis' as a relational concept in different situations. It lies in contrast to the observational and probabilistic connotations of prognosis. The stories have provided many open ends for the reader's imagination to expand, and I fully admit that my reading has been flavoured by my aims in the chapter. Time is not easy to grasp, and the ideas that I offer in this first section may therefore likewise be difficult to grasp. I present them to suggest how the daily practice of the physician can be illuminated within the context of some philosophical ideas, in the hope that you may be inspired to follow them up.

The two sections of the chapter are written as a whole but are still partly independent. The reader, who hesitates at reading a text inspired by philosophy, may nevertheless get something out of the chapter by starting from the section entitled 'When the future overrules the present'.

The world

Intuitively we grasp that, if time could actually stop, there would be nothing at all. Time is essential to our perception of reality. Things change, move, disappear and return. The cycles of nature become the rhythms of human cultures. It is not easy to conceive of this 'nothing' as given to experience, and not just as the logical opposite of 'something'. The mind halts at the fringe of the incomprehensible. However, at its outlook the intuition of 'nothing at all' is not logical. The world has an impact on us even between the reaches of concepts, an impact to which we cannot help but respond.

Time and world are one; the real is only 'now', at the instant of its existing. The totality is also the instant, as there is nothing else to embrace it. Time is therefore the continuous becoming of the world, while the world as given is the echo of itself. The historical building discloses the double life of any material item – becoming and withdrawing in the same present. Extended time has to relate to something and is therefore dividing. Eons have their geological anchorages just as the historical époques have their geopolitical and cultural ones, and as the life of a human being has its biographical ones. In disease, time has its anchorage in the biology of the body, which partly determines the prognosis. Without the perception of determination to any degree, prognosis makes no sense.

An echo is a sound separated from its source in and through time. The sound is real, but at the moment of hearing it the source may no longer be there. When we hear the last beat of a distant hammer, the nail is already in place. The echo is the past as present. The patient making a control visit in the final stage of a disease is both his present, and the echo of his healthy days.

In Kant's thinking time is a priori – a knowing that is independent, or before, experience. Time is an invention of mind that in its very creation unites mind and world[1] in a way that makes sense of experience. Although a priori, time also satisfies the social and scientific needs of chronology. What time is it? As the fourth dimension, time makes it possible to apply mathematics to experience, and thus, to approach the world technologically.

Causality is the time dimension of the world as grasped by humans.[2] The line binding 'recent', 'now' and 'soon' together is rather straight. Most of our expectations for the near future are reasonable; the sun will rise tomorrow, and the oceans persist. Any singular causality rests on, or links up with, other causalities. When we speak of the empirical world, causality is its limit. Since time is the becoming of the world, neither standing still nor going backward are options; true permanence is a perceptual illusion. Causality necessarily entails change; the cause of something past becoming the present, or of something present becoming its future. Since the world is a world of causality and causalities, change is that which brings about the permanence of the world as world. Causality is then permanence through change. The steady ground under our feet is the acceleration of the universe. Health is continuous adaption rather than steady state.

Life establishes a relative freedom within causality. Evolution is its jumps and breaks. The genetic code lays the unreliable pattern of the free will. Subjectivity is the highest form of relative freedom within causality. In action it intervenes in that same causality from which it was born. As a vague contour, one may discern a human hand in the eye of the cyclone. Or perhaps causality is merely devouring the products of human arrogance.

The body is both subjectivity and causality; both the experience and the experienced; both me and my world.[3] In the predictable trajectory of a defined disease the prognosis expresses the causality of the body as nature. Or, to be more precise, the disease is nature by virtue of its causality. Treatment opens new directions in causality; it changes the course of disease. Through medicine humanity manipulates its own collective body – its shadow in causality – with ever-increasing energy and resolution. There is no predefined limit to this project. Whenever patients receive successful up-to-date treatments, the causality of the collective body is modified in ways that may take generations to take effect. The moments of discovery of past scientists will by then be unintelligible, invisible or forgotten. Fate has been rewritten but not outrun. In causality there is only relative freedom, and there will always be prognosis.

Experience

Real time, the continuous becoming of a 'now' dwelling in eternity, is not really experiential, but rather inferred. It does not stand out as an object of consciousness because it exists within everything there is. It is given-with as the universal horizon of experience. The present as a stream of consciousness in which the world is apprehended as a world of time, does however not manage without past and future.[4] Like the musical phrase that needs some degree of extension to transcend from sound to music, the present needs extension to make sense and images of the appearances of the world. Past, present and future are aspects of time by virtue of the distinctions between them, and through which they refer to one another. The past develops as the disappearance of the present; it is what it is by being gone. The future is the projection of causality; it is what it is by being the continuing promise of devouring the present and leaving it over to the past. It is the realisation of everything in the ever-vanishing present.

The present is not just that which differs from past and future; it even actually contains them.[5] This is what gives the necessary extension. The echo or 'retention' of the immediate past also bears the anticipation of an immediate future – the 'protention', and in this fusion the very 'now' is lost. Only in its being asynchronous with the world, consciousness gets sight of it. We are all lost in this translation.

Being and time – Martin Heidegger

Only the living ceases to live. Non-living things cannot die; they can only cease to exist, vanish or become transformed. The existence of the living is an issue also to itself. Reproduction in a wide sense is what the worldly life is about. The 'freedom' of the hawk in the sky is freedom only to the human eye, ignoring the bird's unceasing instinct to catch its prey. For Martin Heidegger,[6] becoming aware of one's existence in its naked form as simply being is not the knowing *of* something like an object, but a disclosure that is a disclosure of itself – *Dasein*. Ultimately, what here is understood is finitude. Being is futural and it is through its temporalisation that existence is laid bare to itself. To face the future resolutely, even though this future is ultimately about death, is to accept a present from which being can be ahead of itself, and a past of factual circumstances, from which the present continuously departs. But this threefold temporality is not extended. With varying emphasis it pertains to being at any instant and in any existential involvement.

Since being is 'being in the world' all phenomena of the world are disclosed along with being through temporality. Primarily, objects are not known in the cognitive sense but partake in existence; they are lived. The time of narration and history, and even the inner time as laid out by Husserl, are abstractions from the temporality of being. The fact that *Dasein* is its own disclosure or understanding implies that it is mostly hidden from itself in the course of our everyday involvement with the social and material world. Authenticity does not prevail but is always a possibility. As such it is the foundation of living and experiencing. Even when hidden by distraction or fear, authenticity is still the central issue – a case of being hiding itself from its own understanding.

Anxiety, fear without an object, is the state of mind that discloses being. When awareness of disease imposes an actual or believed threat to life as hitherto lived, the disclosure of being is close, but being so it is also feared. The fear of the disease is then the fear of the concrete details of the prognosis, but also the fear of the anxiety in face of the future as finitude. This struggle moves the doctor into commitment to the patient; moments of disclosure make up the being of their relationship.

Time and otherwise than being – Emmanuel Levinas

To Emmanuel Levinas,[7] first a pupil and then harsh critic of Heidegger, time is diachronic. This means that it is, from a stance in the present, both that from which individual and collective experience is ordered into past, present and future, and the absolute loss of that which has passed. Levinas points out that an event can never be reduced to a present moment since, by the time consciousness grasps it, it has already passed. In the latter sense continuity between past and present does not exist; the past we talk about is 'pre-original' or 'foreign to every present'. There is no gradient from the recent to the distant, or even archaic. It is time as 'otherwise than being' in which nothing exists or can be represented. Diachrony installs a difference in the identical, at any time the enigma of that which is given. There is the experience of the world as well as its tacit 'echo', the latter being hither to the present. Memory conceals the radical difference through its very function. Yesterday was yesterday as last year was last year; everybody would agree. But where and what yesterday is, is not possible to state, and in relation to immediate and practical needs in human life this question may not even seem relevant. But to Levinas, to disregard the fact that the question has no answer, is to be blind to the limits of reason. Totality and infinity are not the same.[8] Like the vanishing of time, infinity offers no answer; time disappears into infinity.

The irreversible loss through time includes subjectivity. When it takes hold of its present as a human 'being' something is already lost. Time and subjectivity do not coincide. The retention of the immediate past appears to repair the break, but still the break holds the incommensurability of the being of phenomena and concepts, and the beyond being of the past. The residue of the diachrony in subjectivity is sensitivity to the signal of infinity that also is the equivocality of experience. As opposed to Heidegger who, in the impersonal *Dasein*, sees a subjectivity that basically understands its being in the world, Levinas sees the designation of subjectivity as the loss of itself in diachrony and the substitution of oneself for another. There is a craving for the other, not in the sense that the other may satisfy my needs, and thereby restore my lost self, but the reverse; I have an unconditional responsibility for the other even before I have met him. The signal or echo from the pre-original past is the face of the other. Its nakedness and vulnerability is a command. I respond before any present, in passivity, 'as though the invisible that bypassed the present left a trace just by bypassing the present'. Here is the origin of morality and commitment. Meeting the eyes of the other, in the depth of my responsibility, gives no other choice than making him my neighbour. The 'otherwise than being' is the Good.

Why the face? The face is an expression; it is always saying something. Saying is the verb form of language, and in the creation of references, it is both the said and the unsayable. It is an effort through which the unsayable is betrayed, and the said forms knowledge, language, propositions, theory and so forth. The unsayable is expressed in the face and received in sensibility but not understood, being pre-original and otherwise than being. It is the trace left by the invisible. Time unfolds as diachrony, and with an ethical designation, in front of the other.

Within a Levinasian perspective, the doctor is committed already, before the patient who is to receive his or her prognosis enters the consulting room. Time unfolds within this commitment, rather than the commitment arising in face of the patient's anticipated future. The medical encounter gives certain clarity to subjectivity as losing oneself – one's interests – in front of the other. Explicit medical ethics is commensurable with Levinasian ethics, although it resides within a humanism that does not go beyond established worldviews. The 'otherwise than being' presupposes a world in which it is invisible. Therefore, the particulars are still very relevant. The individual biography and future of the patient, and the drama of the existential disclosure, all draw the doctor into moral and empathic engagement. The fact that Levinas contests Heidegger as regards the founding of subjectivity, needs not be a problem to this chapter. As a knowing of man, Heidegger's philosophy still has a lot to tell.

When the future overrules the present

Any symptom or illness has its prognosis – its future – but this fact is not always an issue within the doctor–patient interaction. In the case of most short-lived illnesses, the prognosis is one of the main characteristics of the disease itself – limited duration, complete recovery, usually without treatment. The disease is also its course. There is the mutual trust that the illness will heal, with or without treatment. Nevertheless, preoccupation with the present may be intense and troubled and in really serious situations, the loss of the future has yet other implications. As Martyn Evans has pointed out, in Volume one of this series, the demands of the present moment may prevent us from seeing more than a few days, or even hours, ahead.[9] In the intensive care units (ICUs) doctors and nurses do their best to support people to stay alive rather than preventing them from dying.

When the focus is that of a longer-term prognosis, the future seems, at least temporarily, important and dense, and tends to overrule the present. The present, as it exists at the moment of informing the patient about the result of an examination, assumes significance as the moment of forecast.

Whether or not the prognosis is discussed explicitly in any specific encounter is not an immediate measure of its importance. The doctor's decisions about how to explain the prognosis may pose considerable challenges to professional judgement and sensibility, a struggle of which the patient is usually unaware. If it emerges that a patient has very definite ideas or beliefs about the future, and the doctor does not share those ideas and beliefs, things are liable to go wrong, as Jill Gordon points out in Chapter 7.

A prognosis connotes a forecast, where the bearer of time is disease – confirmed, suspected or feared. It is the disease as future. In practical terms it is first and foremost an extrapolation from a given state to an expected disease state. As for other phenomena, time is subsumed, which in terms of prognosis entails certain complications. When doctor and patient agree to meet again in six months' time, they make a more or less informed jump in their imagination. From a few crucial disease parameters the doctor sketches a reference point with which to compare the future facts. The continuity of the disease process, which is the real disease, then fades from view. This is necessary and inevitable but still it is a loss.

In person-centred care, there is also the prognosis in the sense of the patient himself or herself as future, which (from the shared outlook of patient and doctor) may take precedence over the future course of disease. Continuity of care makes time the editor and makes the patient his or her own personal prognosis.

The biopsychosocial perspective – holistic prognosis

A prognosis is always a prognosis in context. The very course of disease interacts, as an aspect of the patient, with his or her living conditions.[10] This belongs to a branch of epidemiology characterised as biopsychosocial medicine.[11] Agents other than the merely biological or physical have the potential to cause and affect disease.[12] The total number of people, each exposed to, and interacting with, their world, establishes populations at risk. Over time, epidemiological data have become theoretically explained, or anchored in theoretical models that describe the interactions between experience and the body, and within the latter, the interplay between its systems in response to experience.[13] Generally speaking, psychosocial strain of sufficient severity induces a general susceptibility to disease and an increased vulnerability in established disease.[14,15] Biopsychosocial knowledge reminds the doctor to attend to the facts of the patient's life and to bring them into prognostic thinking, a form of probabilistic reasoning. The patient is inversely inferred from epidemiology and theory as a biopsychosocial being, apt to fit into the assessment of risk. The direction of reasoning is from the general to the individual. In the encounter, a holistic prognosis is by necessity impressionistic. It is the imagined result of the interaction of the person with his or her life-conditions and with therapy in a broad sense. Chronic conditions, with or without symptoms, and symptoms due to stress or sensitivity, may add to the whole.

The holistic outlook may lead the doctor to involve other professions in giving social or psychological support, which sometimes makes a difference, both in the present and in the future. In well-defined high-risk situations, such as drug abuse during pregnancy, there may be a need for more elaborated programmes. This is as far as scientific medicine will reach, but, of course, medicine is a lot more than its science. Within the biopsychosocial domain, science is but a framework; clinical medicine's practice, actions and relations are what really count. In terms of prognosis, the difference is that between the judgement of risk and the anxiety felt when standing beside the patient trying to discern his or her future. It is here that the biopsychosocial being turns into a person.

Personal prognosis

From most consultations, people leave with the explicit or implicit message that they will manage. In the context of general practice, 'manage' may mean many different things, including a considerable amount of suffering or insecurity. But mostly, the message implies that life will continue more or less normally. When the current symptom is temporary, prognosis may seem too pretentious a word. Symptoms just come and go; if they tend to recur, or to last for too long, this is an insight that can be gained only in retrospect. If there is a prognosis in the GP's mind, it is about the openness of the future and the reasonable guess that the patient will be in good enough shape both next time, and in the years to come: 'See you' is what we unthinkingly say to one another.

Prognosis can be seen as just one version of a person's future as experienced by the doctor from within the relationship. This version of prognosis is based on the doctor's holistic prognosis, but what makes it differ from this is the commitment. Personal prognosis is 'prognosis-in-relation', that is, a prognosis that matters morally to the doctor, and indeed may be affected by the fact that it matters. Personal prognosis includes the long-term contribution of the doctor–patient relationship that, of course, is difficult to discern within the whole. However, at a certain point of time in a person's life the doctor–patient relationship may well be the difference between life and death.

The scientifically flavoured expression 'general susceptibility to disease'[16] may correspond to the personal prognosis in its widest sense; even when no disease exists, it can express the vulnerability that a GP may sense in patients who live under bad socio-economic conditions, or lead lives full of other hardships, or it may just express vulnerability as such. It may also refer to the sense of fate that colours the mood of any consultation; anything may happen to anybody at any time. This very general statement becomes painfully concrete throughout the lifelong learning of a GP. The risk is a calculation of probability of falling ill or dying within a defined interval of time. The prognosis includes the steps and stages and passages that, in containing time, build up continuity. In retrospect, the prognosis is always inevitable. This corresponds with literary form – a story that begins with the end, or builds it in as a tragic expectation. As the emotion of loss, grief embodies the passing of time in the text that makes it find its way into the reader's own life. Through the form of reversed time, free will turns into causality and determination and loss. The dramatic moments, such as when called to a patient's home to verify his or her death, or when really suddenly realising that a child has been abused, create a heightened attentiveness in the GP, responding to the general susceptibility of patients. The GP is a reader of the prognoses of her or his patients from endpoints that have not yet occurred.

When time stops

Often patients imagine the worst when unknown symptoms arise. Their own prognoses are the immediate reflections of their fear – emotions that find their resonances in cognition. Fear amplifies the experience but usually, on these occasions, the doctor realises very quickly that the patient is basically healthy, and the doctor is able to communicate this to the patient, even before a proper problem definition has been made. But from time to time, the benign epidemiology of primary care, suggesting the presupposition of the common in common symptoms, has to be suspended. The ominous weight and clarity of the patient's story is sometimes enough. At other times the patient knows that something is very wrong, although the symptoms and signs are not specific. Here, the peripeteia of the consultation may develop slowly in a reluctance to acknowledge what is already known. On yet other occasions, a test or examination ordered 'to be on the safe side' results in the unexpected. Irresistibly, the words describing the facts of the body are waiting to be pronounced and in the moments of their preparation, time stops. Nothing real can be done until the new situation is shared and named. Very concretely the future has become a menace, and in being so it takes up all of our attention. It takes precedence over the present. The office where doctor and patient meet becomes a vehicle of sudden loneliness. Patients are friends, but a special kind of friends, with the practice mostly being the only location of the relationship. Still, in certain respects, they may be even closer than the doctor's own family. The straightness of the conversations in a GP's practice is often striking. Matters are addressed that patients hesitate to bring up even with their spouses. Such a context-bound straightness and friendliness is usually the contract and the background of the interaction, but in the moment of naming the threat, the relationship is really tested. The doctor gives voice to merciless nature, and unwillingness to take on this task may cause tense and ambiguous talk, perceived by the patient as distance. The doctor is also lonely in this moment, but nonetheless responsible for restoring the present, which is that relationship entered only by a commitment that seems momentarily lost. Two things may be done to break this vicious circle. First, the doctor can recall that the truth of nature is part of the commitment. Causality is no less human than subjectivity. Tension and ambiguity in giving the probable prognosis to the patient is matched by the strength of the commitment. Just talking, as if nothing had changed, would be the real offence. The felt distance is a message that the doctor is on the right moral track. Overcoming the distance, still remembering the purpose of the relationship, leads to a revised contract with the patient in his or her new and difficult predicament. Second, eyes and faces bear human relationships.[17] If the doctor manages to respond to the patient's look, overcoming the regret of having brought bad news, this may bring the patient back from a chaotic future, to become present. This, in turn, may help the doctor to become a companion again.

When life ends

When a person is close to death, the specific disease steps back. Death does not ask for diagnoses. Everything is about time, in which the dying person is embodying its passage. Dying is the expansion of death in the living – first as the increasing faintness of the physiology of the body and then as the actual death of tissue. Through the increasing coldness of his hands, the patient takes farewell of his doctor. In registering this, the doctor takes farewell of the patient. Disintegrating causality defines the final stage of their relation. Sooner or later, the eyes are no longer there to be met.

The prognosis of the dying person is death. There is no future other than in a strictly chronological sense. Instead, all that remains is an extended present that is the anticipation of its own ending. Depending on its actual duration, and on the degree of unrest and suffering, this present becomes extended also in the perception of those who are companions on the journey. The doctor's commitment does not weaken with the loss of vitality of the patient. Stepping into the bedroom of a dying patient at any stage demands immediate respect. Serenity prevails, even though there may be a struggle going on. The past of the doctor–patient relationship, perhaps even a shared decision and sensitivity to the wordless wishes of the patient, decides whether mitigating arrangements should be made; to bypass dying by means of sedation is always a serious decision.

When the patient has died, the body still belongs to the present. Like an echo it is the remaining matter of the person who was recently alive. It is as real as the person is unreal. On the other hand, the impact of the life of the person, and the network of his or her relations, is still out there among the others. This is not an echo. It is rather the person, freed of matter, but as unforeseeable future.

THE STORIES

Rachel

When Rachel appears in this book series for the first time it is after falling into a diabetic coma behind the closed door of the toilet in her home. This is the way her life with diabetes starts. What happens to her has as yet no name. In the second volume, she lies in her bed in the ward, trying to grasp and face the facts of the disease, and to make out her very first ideas about what her life will be like, being a 'diabetic'. When diabetes first hits her (although at the time it had no other name than thirst, running to the toilet and increasing fatigue) the prognosis does not belong to any taxonomy. All that which is done and said by the doctors and nurses has a back that is invisible to them but that is active in Rachel's life. In her experience of professional interventions one senses fear and rebellion mixed with the instinct for self-preservation and the wish to find some bright sides to her situation. The seriousness of the long-term prognosis is far out of sight. The immediacy of the needles is much more frightening. Later it appears that Rachel's mother is stuck in her fear at the diagnosis. This makes diabetic control her main issue. She mixes shame with submission towards the paediatric staff. The preoccupation with the bodily facts and the felt power of medicine hinders her from developing her human motherly relationship as courageously as Rachel probably needs. Dax the diabetic nurse and Aunt Vimal are the ones who, with different prerequisite strengths, provide security and confidence. With better odds, this may have been enough for Rachel to assimilate her diabetes, but, as we shall see when next we meet her, her social exposure outreaches the support that she gets. The needles have a destructive connotation in attracting boys who inject drugs. She feels guilty about the fate of the girl next to her in the ward, who erroneously gets Rachel's insulin injection. She is aware that she has gone astray in her own life; in the epilogue we learn that Rachel is pregnant. Now, the diabetes imposes on her a responsibility for her child, only fifteen years younger than herself.

With the insights that come from a biopsychosocial perspective, the doctors and nurses around Rachel are all aware of the fact that she is a young person at considerable risk.[18] The immediate prognosis is an important issue, both in itself, and as it affects the long-term prognosis. Despite this insight, things go bad. Was this all determined from the start, whatever the professional efforts, or could Rachel's first years as a 'diabetic' have taken another turn? As the story is filtered through Rachel's own perception, there may have been many things done that never come to our knowledge as readers, but if the efforts were extensive they would somehow have appeared in Rachel's story. The only person in the hospital that seems to make a difference to Rachel herself is Dax. They have an obvious rapport. The doctors occupy a background role. Probably Dax realises it all: that the diabetes imposes a distance between Rachel and her mother, who in her fear sees the diabetes before seeing her daughter. The loneliness in the toilet at the outset seems to have a sad prognostic implication. Dax can probably see how Rachel withdraws when testing becomes the whole issue, but she focuses on the mother's worries and questions without really approaching her need for counselling. Dax is experienced. She likes Rachel, and sees the dangers and the possible shadows that are cast across Rachel's future. She is committed, always at hand, but lacks the competence and power necessary to induce change. She is part of an organisation that is incapable of converting her commitment into action in her patient's long-term interest. Hence the organisation is not receptive to the real prognosis, which is Dax's instinct to protect Rachel from the harshness of her future. As Dax's and Rachel's 'present' face to face is mostly occupied by practicalities and by the anxiety of Rachel's mother, it does not open towards the future. Rather, it is repeated, statically.

Beyond the moment in which we finally say goodbye to Rachel, we can only hope that she will somehow maintain a trusting relationship with Dax, or someone like Dax, to help her to manage her diabetes through pregnancy and motherhood – someone who will sense the fragility of her life project in a realistic way.

Jake

In the early part of his story, Jake is freed from his psoriatic isolation by the brave initiative taken by his girlfriend, Carol. Exposing his flaking skin to bodily closeness is both his desire and his dread. But there is also a second medical problem, his irritable bowel. Whereas the skin disease is a troublesome aspect of him, as his interface with the elements and the items of the physical world, and with others, his unreliable gut is an ever-present threat. It is amplified by any nervousness and, in addition, it has spells obviously of its own. This makes him protective. He guards his autonomy by refusing examination of that which impedes his autonomy. While Carol apparently passes over the threshold of his skin integrity, he will allow no one, after the unexpected proctoscopy described in Volume two, to look into his lower interior again, nor even mention it. Even Carol is excluded, with catastrophic results. So even if the psoriasis is in focus where Jake's story ends it was not the cause of his break up with Carol. On the contrary, as a couple, Jake really felt 'she saw him, not the psoriasis'. He preserves her accepting hands, and his own love, with the tube of hand-cream of a brand originally chosen by Carol. The drawer of his office desk holds a secret that holds his life together.

In terms of Jake's holistic prognosis, the building and breaking of his relationship with Carol are probably crucial. Psoriasis interacts with psychosocial stress,[19] and irritable bowel syndrome (IBS) is recognised as multifactorial with an important relationship with psychosocial circumstances. [20] The one doctor we meet is the GP, Dr Siddha, who is correctly concentrating on the blood in the stools, but who never widens the perspective on Jake's situation beyond the proctoscope. Even so, a formal psychosocial history would most probably have provided only a meagre understanding of Jake's burning predicament. Even as a doctor one has to get under his skin. This may happen only by Jake's implicit invitation, which in turn will be given only if asked for very convincingly. We are not here talking about arguments but about the doctor's open interest in what will happen to Jake in the hours immediately after the consultations, and then in the days, weeks and years ahead. It is not just curiosity about what may lie around the corner for Jake. It is the moral commitment of the personal prognosis, which in itself contains time, when Jake and the doctor meet in a relationship that reaches far beyond what they each can grasp.[21] In this space,

Jake's bodily reality and desperate self-fulfilling loneliness are captured in the imagined consultation occurring at the time of his break-up with Carol.[22] His medical conditions and his loneliness are no longer his alone, but become shared in the 'cool intimacy' of the doctor–patient relationship.[23] If such sharing can happen, and can be accompanied by trust, perhaps Jake will have less to hide from Carol. This could alter his future in fundamental ways, including the pattern that we understand to be his prognosis.

Liz

Life happens to Liz. She is usually a bit late, rushing and hot, trying to catch up. Reminded by a daily anti-epileptic pill, she lives at the horizon of the unknown and uncontrolled within herself. She is a wakeful sensor of her own consciousness, always slightly distracted. It is not just the fits; there is the aura and the aftermath – a mental haze with loss of words, memory and orientation in space. Shame is a feeling that generalises into a mood, colouring a lot more than her imagined being, exposed and helpless during the seizures. Fear prevents her from building proactive psychological defences. Threats appear indiscriminately and safeguarding her integrity is all important. Her daughter, Sophie, gently grounds her, and seems to be able to combine being a child with family responsibility. They are a good team. We know nothing about Liz's love life, but we do discover, in the last part of her story, that she would like to become pregnant again.

Although a stranger, the epilepsy is part of Liz. To try to discern its prognosis as a strand of its own in Liz's overall future is not very meaningful. And – to complicate matters – there are other prognoses. In the story of the second volume, she receives a letter informing her that the smear shows cervical dysplasia. For Liz, the news carries the implications of cancer and death. A few stark words in print and the present is invaded by the future. Standing at the airport with Sophie, waiting for departure, she manages to contact her GP, Dr Wocjik, over the phone. Dr Wocjik knows Liz, and understands immediately the dark imaginings making up the contours of Liz's own prognosis. Here the personal prognosis, the 'prognosis-in relation', is dictated by Liz's experience. What the doctor does is stronger than just giving the reassuring probabilistic facts. She understands the drama, but keeps her mind clear. The defencelessness of Liz's personality enforces the doctor's commitment, and makes her add paternalism in a carefully weighed dosage. Over the years, doctor–patient contacts like this one may actually alter Liz's 'real' medical prognosis. Confidence, comfort and other outcomes of consultations may lower her level of stress, in turn shown to raise the seizure threshold.[24] However, again, mere knowledge about the psychological triggers and their prevention, and its correct implementation in the clinic, would not lead Dr Wocjik to imagine Liz where she was standing at the airport.

The 'prognosis' of a possible pregnancy is the theme in Liz's story in this final volume. Here Liz encounters a gynaecologist who has limited knowledge about her context and biography, but she obviously becomes committed. Although the 'real' consultation is passed, she invites Liz for a second consultation about her considered pregnancy. A benevolent paternalistic or maternalistic impulse awakens. From all the 'buts' we have to conclude that the doctor feels that a pregnancy may not be very wise. Obviously the concerns are primarily about the baby, but behind that may lie a thought that giving birth to a second child may not be the best thing for Liz either. This has to be an intuition of hers, very close to a prejudice, but perhaps she is struck by the certain vulnerability in Liz's personality. So there is a personal prognosis growing within the relationship and it deals with both the possible mother and the possible baby. As with the experience of cervical dysplasia, the imagined future is more powerful than the present facts. In fact, we do not know how seriously Liz is considering a pregnancy. Maybe the most important thing is simply knowing that she has a choice once again.

In spite of the gynaecologist's good intentions, her conversation with Liz does not come out well. The failure is not repaired by the small talk about Sophie at the end. The doctor's original concern for the patient is captured by her formal agenda.[25] Liz never gets the opportunity to talk about her wish to become pregnant. If, for instance, there is no defined father – there is no 'we' in Liz's question to the doctor, or later on the Internet site – and she feels safe enough to talk about this, the conversation may take another direction. We can imagine that Dr Wocjik in this situation would have been able to invite Liz to talk about being a woman of 38 years, with epilepsy, and being on a potentially teratogenic drug, with the fits never far away, a mother of a talented daughter but with little success in establishing sustainable relations with men, and the years just passing. Dr Wocjik would then perhaps think that precisely the vulnerability that makes her so committed to Liz may keep too many men away. She cannot explain to herself why this is so, nor what it is that makes her so committed. A moment of silent sadness is shared. And then up to the surface again, saying goodbye, the doctor following Liz in her thoughts after she closes the door and walks down the corridor towards her future. And, maybe, Liz here tries on the thought that there will be a life for her whether or not there are any more babies. Or maybe she does not.

Jen and Geoff

The fates of Jen and Geoff are intertwined, even after Jen has died. They were not quite that young when they met, both having been married before, but as Jen's twin sister Jane puts it, 'It had always been true love. Unmitigated.' Jane was not happy about their marriage because she partly lost Jen. Geoff's daughter Mary felt abandoned when her father far too quickly, in her opinion, remarried. So in choosing each other, Jen and Geoff seem to have departed from the safe shores of social conventions and security. They did everything together. Jen kept on choosing Geoff, unconditionally, even when he suffered a stroke with ensuing hemiplegia and a change of personality, becoming difficult to live with and immensely dependent.

When we get to know them, Jen, being a smoker, is losing weight, lacking in energy and is coughing blood. Dr Gaitens, their GP, strongly suspects lung cancer. Jen's major concern is Geoff, and when she is in hospital to be investigated, he falls deeper into his depression and needs care. He is practically non-communicative, other than the glint in his eyes when Jen comes to see him and the change in mood when she leaves. Without antidepressants he would probably have starved to death.

Jen dies in torment, at a period of time after chemotherapy that we do not know, and thereafter Geoff lives on in total inwardness in the ward. Five years after Jen's death, Jane writes a letter to Mary to ask her to 'let nature take its course', but from the letter one understands that Mary, in weekly telephone calls, chases the staff to do everything to keep her father alive.

The pattern of the final years for Jen and Geoff is firmly laid, in the causality of nature, in their bodies and in the tightness of the bonds between them. Dr Gaitens is a witness, and he has access to the hospital and the elderly care home, but had he not opened these doors then someone else must have done that. The effects on Geoff of losing Jen – his ensuing existential suffering – would lie open to the experienced doctor as part of his prognosis. There were no alternatives. Seeing these effects need not cause disillusionment and pessimism; on the contrary, it is the basis of empathy. Dr Gaitens is sensitive to the shift in Geoff's mood in the early stage of Jen's disease. But his compassion and commitment as such do not appear to offer much by way of support to the old lovers. Their little system is mainly self-sustaining. In this situation, the doctor's compassion is most important to himself, supporting him to keep his ardour as a doctor through all of the suffering that he still has to encounter through his career.

Chemotherapy is the recommended treatment in small-cell lung cancer, on average increasing the life-expectancy, whether the cancer is contained or has spread, but deaths from treatment also occur.[26] Maybe it gave Jen (and Geoff) some respite, but one does not get the impression that they were able to spend more time together in their home, something that would have been the ultimate criterion of an improved prognosis. If involved in the discussions about the pros and cons of treatment, Dr Gaitens would surely have been sceptical if chemotherapy would not bring about any increased probability for Jen and Geoff to return home. But it is quite likely that the doctor's doubts about the benefit of treatment would have been overruled by Jen herself, who would accept any treatment that, to any extent, in her own imagination, may give her more time with Geoff.

The final prognostic issue in the lives of Jen and Geoff is, at least theoretically, the conflict between life-expectancy and quality of life during Geoff's final years. His daughter Mary, from a distance, wants him to stay in her life as long as possible, and urges the staff to put him under all kinds of treatment, resuscitation included. Although the actual outcome of these efforts can hardly be a prolongation of meaningful life, Mary's demands make Jane spell out the imminent dilemma of medicine in situations where death is reasonably close. In her letter, concluding the stories of this book series, she is the one to make the personal prognosis based on her unconditional commitment to Geoff, the man who once, more or less, took her twin sister away from her, and who hits out at her when she comes to visit him. She has the gift of altruism and senses how he suffers in an eternal present, where death is the only future and the only rescue.

THE CONSULTATION – DETERMINATION AND OPENNESS

When the patient departs into the corridor, and then into the outside street, carrying the doctor's implicitly made prognosis as a lasting mood and memory from the interaction, he or she is at every instant embodying and capturing the prognosis, from short term to long term. This goes on and on until the next visit, or until something happens that breaks the curve of anticipation. The older or more fragile the patient is, the wider the spread of probable outcomes at a future point of time. In this broad sense, in its longest term, the prognosis is one and the same for everyone. To claim a certain specificity, the personal prognosis we are here talking about, does not aim quite so far into the future. The doctor needs the ability to make an intermediate judgement; he or she needs to ask, 'How are things going?' and he or she needs to do so with an emphasis that extends the phrase beyond the banality of merely chatting and invites from the patient an honest response. That is, 'How are things *really* going?' is what the patient needs to perceive in the question, in order to be encouraged to investigate his or her version of the human condition. Here, prognosis retains its meaning only when it is converted into a GP's continuing attention. The personal prognosis is, as noted, a relational concept. It is established continuously through a chain of encounters, where doctor and patient look into the past of the patient to think about the future. Nothing in what has happened can be changed or undone. In the strictly temporal aspect all is determined up to the point of the conversation. Resolutions that failed, things that were not said, small but pivotal choices, births and deaths and the winds of society are all the stern facts of the past. Of all possible trajectories this is the one that actually eventuated. But as a baseline for the future much of what is definite turns into possibilities and perhaps options. In re-presenting the world, the present also questions and challenges it. There is a margin of freedom, variable and individual, within the large movement of the implacable. In suddenly opening spaces within the present, doctor and patient may in interaction intervene in the patient's future. It may be an agreed decision but it may simply be recognition of the inevitable – eyes that meet and with that meeting convey a message from doctor to patient about human dignity. Hope and intentions may then slightly increase the ratio in the prognosis between contingency and determination.

Like poetry the margin of freedom may have deep implications for the future, without clear indications of what these implications may be. Still, when the prognosis within the everyday ritual of the consulting room discloses time, the tension of the fleeting present vanishes. The prognosis is no longer only 'then'; it is also the extension of 'now', which means that the relationship, and that which has been learned within it, persist. Neither time nor person is cut into pieces of abstraction, and that is why the prognosis, when it is at its most real, it is also at its most personal. The mutuality in the understanding of the patient's past becomes at the same instant the vivid content of the relationship in the present and the possible content of important aspects of the future.

REFERENCES

1. Kant I. *Critique of Pure Reason.* (Trans. M Weigelt). London: Penguin Classics; 2007.
2. Kant I. op.cit.
3. Merleau-Ponty M. *The Phenomenology of Perception.* (Trans. C Smith). London: Routledge & Kegan Paul; 1962.
4. Husserl E. *On the Phenomenology of the Consciousness of Internal Time.* (Trans. J Barnett Brough). Dordrecht: Kluwer Academic Publishers; 1992.
5. Husserl E. op.cit.
6. Heidegger M. *Being and Time* (Trans. J Macquarie and E Robinson). Oxford: Basil Blackwell; 1962.
7. Levinas E. *Otherwise Than Being, or, Beyond Essence.* (Trans. A Lingis). Pittsburgh: Duquesne University Press; 1999a.
8. Levinas E. *Totality and Infinity.* (Trans. A Lingis). Pittsburgh, PA: Duquesne University Press; 1969.
9. Evans M. Music, interrupted: an illness observed from within. In: Evans M, Ahlzén R, Heath I, *et al.*, editors. *Medical Humanities Companion Volume One: symptom.* Oxford: Radcliffe Publishing; 2008. pp. 14–26.
10. Chida Y, Hamer M. An association of adverse psychosocial factors with diabetes mellitus: a meta analytical review of longitudinal cohort studies. *Diabetologia.* 2008; **51**: 2168–78.
11. Engel G. The need for a new medical model. *Science.* 1977; **196**: 129–36.
12. Cassel J. The contribution of the social environment to host resistance. *Am J Epidemiol.* 1976; **104**: 107–23.
13. Getz L, Kirkengen AL, Ulvestad E. The human biology saturated with experience. *Tidskr Norsk Laegeforen.* 2011; **131**: 683–7.

14. Cassel J. op.cit.

15. Kiecolt-Glaser JK. Psychoneuroimmunology psychology's gateway to the biomedical future. *Perspect Psychol Sci.* 2009; **4**: 367–9.

16. Cassel J. op.cit.

17. Levinas E. op. cit. a and op. cit. b.

18. Lewin AB, Heidgerken AD, Williams LB, *et al.* The relation between family factors and diabetes control: the role of diabetes adherence. *J Paediatric Psychology.* 2006; **31**: 174–83.

19. Koo J, Lebwohl A. Psychodermatology: mind and skin connection. *Am Fam Physician.* 2001; **64**: 173–8.

20. Surdea-Blaga T, Baban A, Dumitrascu DL. Psychosocial determinants of irritable bowel syndrome. *World J Gastroenterol.* 2012; **18**: 616–26.

21. Levinas E. op. cit. b.

22. Heath I. *The Mystery of General Practice.* London: Nuffield Provincial Hospitals Trust; 1995.

23. Evans M, Macnaughton J. Intimacy and distance in the clinical examination. In: Ahlzén R, Evans M, Louhiala P, *et al.* editors. *Medical Humanities Companion Volume Two: diagnosis.* Oxford: Radcliffe Publishing; 2010: 89–107.

24. Roth DL, Goode KT, Williams VL, *et al.* Physical exercise, stressful life experience, and depression in adults with epilepsy. *Epilepsia.* 1994; **35**: 1248–55.

25. Stewart M, Belle Brown J, Weston WW, *et al. Patient centred medicine: transforming the clinical method.* Oxford: Radcliffe Publishing; 2003.

26. Simon G, Turrisi A. Management of small-cell lung cancer. ACCP evidence-based clinical practice guidelines. *Chest.* 2007; **132**(3 suppl): 324–39.

5

Acute and chronic

JOHN SAUNDERS

Far from it being true that man and his activity makes the world comprehensible, he is himself the most incomprehensible of all, and drives me relentlessly to the view of the accursedness of all being, a view manifested in so many painful signs in ancient and modern times. It is precisely man who drives me to the final despairing question: Why is there something? Why not nothing?[1]

> O miserable mankind, to what fall
> Degraded, to what wretched state reserved!
> Better end here unborn. Why is life giv'n
> To be thus wrested from us? Rather why
> Obtruded on us thus? Who if we knew
> What we receive, would either not accept
> Life offered, or soon beg to lay it down,
> Glad to be so dismissed in peace. ...
>   Henceforth I fly not death, nor would prolong
> Life much, bent rather how I may be quit
> Fairest and easiest of this cumbrous charge,
> Which I must keep till my appointed day
> Of rend'ring up, and patiently attend
> My dissolution.[2]

> Why was I not still-born,
> Why did I not die when I came out of the womb?
> Why was I ever laid on my mother's knees

or put to suck at her breasts?
Why was I not hidden like an untimely birth,
Like an infant that has not lived to see the light?…

Why should the sufferer be born to see the light?
Why is life given to men who find it so bitter?
They wait for death but it does not come,
they seek it more eagerly than hidden treasure.
They are glad when they reach the tomb,
and when they come to the grave they exult.
Why should a man be born to wander blindly,
hedged in by God on every side?[3]

We live in an age of chronic illness. The postponement of death has created a huge population with chronic illness. Its management has become a key feature of general practice and the source of a host of specialised clinics: diabetes clinics, asthma clinics, hypertension clinics, memory clinics, epilepsy clinics. Instead of reaching our 60s or 70s and then dying relatively rapidly, an increasing number of people decline gradually. The prevalence of Alzheimer's disease, diabetes, degenerative joint disease, chronic cardiac failure and chronic renal disease has risen steeply in the last quarter of a century. Yet it would be foolish to pretend that chronic disease represents anything new in the overall experience of Western man. What has changed are our expectations. We expect not only to live longer but to live in a fitter state. We expect to die after a short illness, rather than undergoing a gradual decline. We feel cheated if illness somehow catches us and leaves us with ongoing disability. It isn't fair.

And our perceptions have changed, too. Objectively, we have never been healthier. Subjectively, disease stalks us around every corner.[4] Convinced that our environment is filthier and less healthy and that our food is less wholesome and our lifestyles are more hazardous we develop an obsession with health and a belief that chronic illness will become our lot unless we consume special diets, exercise and, of course, undergo incessant check-ups.[5] We vilify the smoker, look disdainfully on the obese and disapprove of the anxious. For the profession we have created a 'nice little earner' treating more and more people for less and less benefit for diseases that we have invented: hypercholesterolaemia at minimally raised mean concentrations, hypertension, elevated blood glucose, stress and sexual dysfunction.

The diseases that we may consider under the phrase 'chronic disease' are legion. Some have relatively few consequences day to day – let us say Addison's disease or hypertension; others affect every minute – let us say Alzheimer's disease. How long does a disease have to be in order to be considered chronic? Some would say as little as three months, but for our purposes here, I want to consider chronic diseases that are likely to last a lifetime. Of these, the examples to consider are diseases that are (usually) associated with patients who most people would consider to be fully autonomous and those diseases that are (usually) associated with loss of mental function. Let us say: diabetes in the first group and chronic schizophrenia and Alzheimer's in the second. Each of these is unequivocally chronic, but each one of them has acute phases and complications.

Chronic disease creates difficulties that can be overcome or that can overcome the sufferer. Sometimes the road is easy; sometimes the road is difficult. The metaphors to which we resort as we recount experiences are those of the journey, the search or the pilgrimage. A few examples from different periods: from ancient literature, Morris's re-telling of *Jason and the Argonauts*; Malory's *Le Morte d'Arthur*; Cervantes's *Don Quixote* (when Dr Richard Blackmore asked Sydenham which authors he should read in order to become a good physician, Sydenham recommended Cervantes[6]); Bunyan's *The Pilgrim's Progress*; Coelho's *The Alchemist*; and even Tony Blair's memoir *A Journey*. It would be easy to extend the list. But what is striking is the constancy of the theme of life as a search or journey with difficulties to be overcome. Animals may adapt to this, but only for humans is there authenticity or dignity.

There is nothing in this that is specially related to illness or disability. To be sure, we can construe disability as one of life's trials; and, whatever Aristotle may have said, the desire to understand or the Socratic 'examined life' is not a quest pursued by many. For many people with chronic disease, it is something in the background, something that has to be accommodated and accepted and that has to be managed through routine: taking the tablets, injecting the insulin, attending the doctor and knowing that one is in some way different from many others. But this too depends on the severity of the disease: for the severely disabled, the result is removal from normal society.

Wilfred Owen reflects on the thoughts of the young man disabled by the war injuries that now define him:

> About this time Town used to swing so gay
> When glow-lamps budded in the light blue trees,
> And girls glanced lovelier as the air grew dim,
> In the old times before he threw away his knees.
> Now he will never feel again how slim
> Girls' waists are, or how warm their subtle hands:
> All of them touch him like some queer disease. …
>
> Tonight he noticed how the women's eyes
> Passed from him to the strong men that were whole.

> How cold and late it is! Why don't they come
> And put him to bed? Why don't they come?[7]

We do not want to be defined by chronic illness in this way. In our first story, Rachel's hospitalisation is precipitated by her trying to ignore the fact that she has diabetes: 'She'd been off her head for weeks, careless with her insulin, not paying any attention to the flu, the chest infection. Why should she? Why did she have to be different?' In our second story, Ellie cannot bear to look at Jake because of his skin: '[S]he flinched when she touched him. Her obsessive interest in his symptoms masked disgust.' Both Rachel and Jake struggle to free themselves of the illnesses that, they fear, define them for others.

'Pathography' is the literary form that deals with the experience of disability. Disabled figures often appear in fiction as sinister characters who demonstrate that power is not always lost, even with the severest physical disability. Zola's *Therese Raquin* is a terrifying story of the power of a woman with locked-in syndrome who realises that the couple who are caring for her are responsible for the murder of the husband of one of them and who drives the couple to their graves.

Pathography is also found in the visual arts with innumerable references to the impact of disability. Compare, for example, two pictures by Edvard Munch. In *The Sick Child*[8] we view an acutely ill child. The scene is rendered slightly out of focus by scratched brush strokes, as if viewed through the artist's own tears. On the one hand is the pallid child, lying on a white pillow; on the other is the mother, isolated by the solitary extended hand and the almost unbearable drama of her impotence against the child's suffering and loneliness. Here the 'drama of suffering can be experienced as a quest for meaning, not as a desperate end to life'.[9]

The second picture, *Self Portrait Between the Clock and the Bed*[10] shows the artist as immobile and sick. Here the drama lies in the lack of movement. The subject's gaze is fixed; his arms are motionless at his side; and he waits for nothing except sleep – the bed is at his side – and death. Light and life are behind him: '[T]he image of death is the eternal background of the dance of life.'[11] The dark shadow of the door lies in the background; the tall clock reminds us of passing time. The figure, like so many who are chronically ill, waits on the threshold. Chronic illness raises questions about the intimacy of character, its strengths and values – qualities that are largely irrelevant to an acute attack of, say, influenza. Such features are beyond rational proof, and identifiable only by an empathic indwelling. In the long journey of chronic disease, character is our innermost resource, our judge or our enemy.

Before leaving this reflection on the visual arts, let me turn to Caspar David Friedrich's masterpiece: *Woman At the Window (Frau am Fenster)*.[12] What could be simpler? Ignore for a moment the subtleties of colour and consider the structure. Inside is the dark, which we enter in a geometric grid of lines from the floor, the windows and the walls. Humanity's aspirations are not limited by this grid. The artist's wife, Caroline, is seen to be looking out of the window of the austere room – her back to the darkness, into light, where the mast of a ship offers an unspecified voyage. Like all window pictures of this period, the image conveys a sense of hope and longing.[13] It is *sehnsucht*, that is, a yearning for the infinite.

The same romanticism inhabits the simple piece of music known to every young pianist, Schumann's *Dreaming*,[14] and Shostakovich's viola sonata can be experienced as a call to transcend chronic illness. He completed it only a month before his death, despite heart failure, cancer, arthritis and failing eyesight, creating a sense of resignation mixed with serenity.[15]

The theme of hope for something unspecified in the onward progression of chronic illness is the subject of Buchan's advice in his essay 'Of the Passions':[16]

> A custom has long prevailed among physicians, of prognosticating, as they call it, the patient's fate, or foretelling the issue of the disease. Vanity no doubt introduced this practice, and still supports it. … I have known a physician barbarous enough to boast, that he pronounced more sentences than all his Majesty's judges. … A friend, or even a physician, may often do more good by a mild and sympathizing behaviour than by medicine, and should never neglect to administer that greatest of all cordials, HOPE.

Within the field of literature, especially the novel, the effects of chronic illness are described in terms of individual experience in a way that no scientific study, with its emphasis on the accumulated experience of groups, can do. The essential facts of diabetic complications are based on population studies; effective healthcare for individuals requires the use of imagination in order to understand the effects of living with a chronic disease on each unique person who is living with a chronic disease. But what does 'effective care' mean? What is the quest, the search, the journey, the pilgrimage actually for? Further, to pursue the ethical question, what should it be for? What choices are permissible in a modern liberal secular democracy? We are brought to the fundamental questions with which this chapter opened: Why life? What for?

But I want to pursue a different line of thought, the contrast between the care of acute and chronic illness, because it throws up the most searching value questions of short- versus long-term gain. Assume for a moment the caricature of a 20-year old with insulin dependent diabetes. What counts for him or her as good quality of life *today* may mean ignoring medical advice, apart from mostly (but not always) giving the insulin. Testing, meals, follow-up clinics and the rest of the paraphernalia are a nuisance that can be ignored: they impact adversely on everyday life. At the age of 20, one is immortal and the doctor's advice against risk-taking is an invitation to take risks. Parents can be ignored. Friends aren't bothered and being the same as them is more important than most things. Taking risks is what being 20 is all about, in our caricature's opinion. The heavy burden of solemn healthcarers intoning the litany of disasters to come is best ignored: it may never happen; it's a chance to be taken. Perhaps it won't be so bad if things go wrong, and treatments will be better in the future. Then move the scene forward, like the spirit in *A Christmas Carol*. Now our brave hero is 37, partially sighted, with gangrenous toes, intermittent diarrhoea from neuropathy and a place on the waiting list for dialysis. With this terrible damage to a life that could have been largely free of such complications, many (still) young people have to come to terms with the awful responsibility of having brought this upon themselves. Rachel in our first story weeps, 'If I'd taken better care of myself …'

This scenario is extremely common. The question it throws up is the sort of advice that the doctor or diabetes nurse should give at an earlier stage in the life story. Perhaps 'advice' is the wrong word: strategy may be more useful. Paternalism is a dirty word in medical ethics and yet it seems that some people need protection from themselves; and that autonomy is more than choice based on a factual appreciation of possibilities. How far does the quality of the relationships with those at home, with friends and with healthcarers who are familiar (and not changing every month) become more important than advice about insulin or hypoglycaemia? How is the short term traded off against the medium term (such as accepting an unsatisfactory situation for a time in order to keep the patient attending and relating, and pursuing a gradual policy), or against the long term?

It would be nice to think that we could measure these complex factors with some simple psychological tool, that we could establish attitudes at different points in the life experience of a chronic disease and that we could prescribe the most effective solution for that time of life. However, solutions must be found for individuals whose personal histories and values are subtly but critically different. Life events change us: the loss of a job, a bankruptcy, an acute illness, the death of a friend and/or the infidelities of those we trust. The impact of chronic illness on our lives changes in each phase of life's journey.

At the beginning, it is all so new. We may be shocked at the revelation that we are going to be wrestling with a condition that arrived unexpected, unbidden and undeserved, for the rest of our lives. Yet there is the excitement of the new: so much to learn and supporting experts around us who impress us with their confidence and enthusiasm. Compliance is high. Our medications are regularly taken. The overall control of our disease is as good as it could be. But then we become backsliders. There can soon be the familiarity of the commonplace, and if the routine of daily care does not come to bore us then it may come to create its own resentments. We may soon feel it to be unfair that we have to live with this uninvited illness when others do not. All of these factors may demotivate us.

Why take care when there is a reasonable chance that we will avoid the disasters with which we are threatened? Or perhaps we succumb to the events around us, the personal troubles that arrive to disturb most lives. We retreat into our shells and life becomes clouded and grey, filled with new anxieties that can never be revealed to the healthcarers whose conceit convinces them that they understand us. Sometimes this will progress to a depressive illness or just a dryness that takes the colour out of daily life, like an overexposed photograph or an old, fading sepia image. Always in the background, there is a constant presence, like a demon on our shoulder. Inject the insulin and check the blood glucose and watch the diet. Or inhale the asthma medication and swallow the pills and do the postural drainage. Or avoid the fatty food and do the exercise. There may seem to be a hundred and one constrictions on our freedom. Can this really be what life is for?

And as we grow older we may seek the narrative or the meaning of our 'journey', the continuities, the wish that the past may have been something more vital and abiding than a wastepaper basket into which our shredded hopes are being deposited. But the concept of life as narrative into which our experience of chronic disease must be somehow forced is not shared by all. For some there is no sense of narrative at all, with or without chronic illness. Life is lived day by day.[17]

Talk of narrative is fashionable. Its central idea is that some of us see our lives as a narrative, a story or series of stories, in which we play a part. We are all actors in our own dramas, played out on the theatre of the world. It is merely a description, an empirical assertion about how we live our lives. This has been called the psychological narrativity thesis: '[S]elf is a perpetually rewritten story. … [I]n the end we become the autobiographical narratives by which we "tell about" our lives.'[18] Many doctors, however, have been sceptical about stories. Patients' stories change on repetition and are interpreted by the time, place and culture in which they are embedded.[19] They can be mistaken, inaccurate, untrustworthy or dishonest. Stohlberg[20] writes:

> Today hardly anyone will seriously assert that man's natural, biological condition can be described independently of existing cultural and linguistic categories or deny that even elementary, seemingly natural bodily phenomena, such as pain, are culturally framed to a high degree.

He goes on to assert that biological processes in the body are grasped only through the language, images and notion of our culture. For him we find ourselves between cultural relativism and static biological essentialism. Corporality and body experience are fundamentally tied to a cultural and historical context – and some crucial aspects vary little across cultures. We communicate with tears.

The storyteller is the expert, but the story must be interpreted, as all history must, and it must not always be accepted as a literal recounting of events. In chronic illness this gives a privileged place to the patient that does not exist in the same way when we develop flu; the context is so much more important in chronic illness. In acute illness a return to normal is possible; in chronic illness, life is irreversibly changed. In that irreversibly changed life, the good doctor sees the 'person in the patient', and not just the patient.[21]

In many Western countries, expenditure on chronic illness takes up two-thirds or more of healthcare budgets. Holman[22] writes that, while variation in patterns of illness creates uncertainty, patients often detect the trends better than their doctors do – if only because the patient is living with his or her own illness. Doctors may have much to offer on specifics, but patients do better when they are partners and not customers. Satisfaction and compliance are better and costs lower. A model that promotes involved understanding offers more than managerialism and endless organisational 'reforms'. It would be nice to add 'continuity of care' to these desirables, since it aids the healing relationship and promotes efficiency. Alas, in many countries this has been largely lost. Patients are associated with practices or they see a member of a specialist team, not an individual doctor. Self-management is inevitable: patients have to do it, day by day. They can and do veto professionals' recommendations. In the partnership paradigm, doctors are experts on disease; patients are expert on their own lives.[23] Both are caregivers. Both are experts. Both determine goals. Motivation is boosted by a shared understanding. We call it 'empowerment' through collaborative education. Advocates of empowerment assert that we have formerly socialised patients into, and fostered, medical dependence in long-term disease management.

This approach sees management as a changing process. In the education of healthcarers there is more to teach than the facts of disease: how to cope with emotional distress, how to communicate, how to manage symptoms and how to establish therapeutic relationships. For this, relevant behavioural sciences are needed to complement the science of disease.[24] However, choice may not be enough. In her monograph, *The Logic Of Care*, Annemarie Mol contrasts the 'logic' of care with the 'logic' of choice. Choice, she says, does not necessarily give better outcomes but may alter daily practices in ways that may not fit well with the intricacies of our diseases. Choice can be manipulated, as every advertiser knows: we can make people long for certain things; and, for care, 'paternal discipline' is needed as well as 'tender love'. Stohlberg comments that capacities and skills may fade in illness. We become 'bafallig' – decrepit in disrepair.

The entire time I was like a drowning person without a rope strong enough to hang on to[25]... Illness turns the body into adversary, a separate existence, (an ontological understanding of illness). It 'had you', weighed on you, clutched you, grabbed you, overcame, struck you, fell upon you, assailed you, or attacked you.

We are not very good at choice. Our choices are clouded by fear, uncertainties, subjective evaluations of particular therapies, excessive confidence or lack of trust in those who advise us and the impossibility of knowing the experience of future states. We may be best being led and, says Mol, focusing on the situations in which choices occur and the activities patients undertake, what they do. Choice sees the individual as a customer; care sees him or her as a sufferer, a patient – and not just an individual but also a member of a collective. In doing things, our choices may change: this is not passivity, but an active engagement between patient and healthcarers that constantly iterates and re-iterates what is needed. There is greater success, higher satisfaction, compliance and continuity of care if each patient is treated as partner. There is good evidence for group visits in which patients set the agenda, as well as the value of self-management information and for remote communication, using the phone, email or text.[26] Moreover, patients often detect the prognostic trends in themselves better, having received the general information from the healthcarer. In healthcare, the patient is one of the producers of health and is not just a consumer; in chronic disease, the principal caregiver.

Years ago a much respected physician, Arnold Bloom, helped to establish diabetes centres and paved the way for shared care and the shift in diabetes practice from hospitals into the community. These are the services that Rachel experiences today. At a meeting on the management of childhood diabetes and how strict standards of control could interfere with a happy childhood, Bloom declared, 'We are all in the happiness business.' But the quest for a perfect ideal of health and happiness is a form of madness,[27] an addiction that can distort our lives. We cannot abolish a chronic disease, as we can an acute one. Each patient lives with it and through it, tempering its miseries with positive experiences and constructive purposes. The journey or pilgrimage will give us no easy answers: we must live with questions.

REFERENCES

1. Schelling FWJ. *Werke.* Schröter M, editor. Munich: Beck; 1927. pp. 13:7.
2. Milton J. *Paradise Lost*; 1667.
3. The Book of Job. **3**; 11–16, 20–3.
4. Barsky AJ. The paradox of health. *New Engl J Med.* 1988; **318**: 414–18.
5. Thomas L. The healthcare system. In: *The Wonderful Mistake: notes of a biology watcher.* Oxford: Oxford University Press; 1988. pp. 176–9.
6. Bamforth I. *The Body In the Library.* Verso; 2002. p. 295.
7. Owen W. *Collected Poems: disability.* London: Chatto & Windus; 1928. P. 67.
8. 1885–86 Oslo: Nasjonalgalleriet.

9. Bordin G, D'Ambrosio LP. *Medicine in Art*. Los Angeles, CA: Getty publications; 2010. p. 314.

10. 1940–43 Oslo: Munch-Museet.

11. Bordin G, D'Ambrosio LP. op. cit. p. 40.

12. 1822 Berlin: Nationalgalerie.

13. Forster-Hahn F, Keisch C. Schuster P-K, *et al. Spirit Of an Age*. London: National Gallery Company; 2001. pp. 70–1.

14. Schumann R. *Kinderscenen*. Op 15; 1844.

15. Shostakovich D. *Sonata for viola and piano*. Op 147; 1975. (O'Neill D. Medical classics. *BMJ*. 2012; **345**: e5860.)

16. Buchan W. *Domestic Medicine: or, a Treatise On the Prevention and Cure of Diseases*. Edinburgh: Balfour & Creech; 1788. p. 128.

17. Strawson G. Against narrativity. *Ratio*; 2004; XVII: 0034–0006.

18. Bruner J. Life as narrative. *Social Research*. 1987; **54**: 11–32.

19. Shapiro J. Illness narrative: reliability, authenticity and the empathic witness. *Med Hum*. 2011; **37**: 68–72.

20. Stohlberg M. *Experiencing Illness and the Sick Body In Early Modern Europe*. Basingstoke: Palgrave Macmillan; 2011. p. 8.

21. Lapsley. *BMJ*. 2012.

22. Holman H. Patients as partners in managing chronic disease. *BMJ*. 2000; **320**: 526.

23. Bodenheimer T, Lorig K, Holman H, *et al*. Patient self management of chronic disease in primary care. *JAMA*. 2002; **288**: 2469–75.

24. Holman H. Chronic disease – the need for a new clinical education. *JAMA*. 2004; **292**; 1057–9.

25. Stohlberg. op. cit. p. 24.

26. H Holman, Lorig K. Patients as partners in managing chronic disease. *BMJ*. 2000; **320**: 526.

27. Greaves D. The obsessive pursuit of health and happiness. *BMJ*. 2000; **321**: 1576.

6

Becoming

JANE MACNAUGHTON

WHAT HAPPENS NEXT? BEING ABLE AND BEING UNABLE

In 2012, the UK was enraptured with Olympic fever and the response to the achievements of able-bodied athletes was far surpassed by watching the extraordinary feats of the paralympians. Martine Wright, the Team GB sitting volleyball athlete who lost both legs in the 7/7 bombings in London, was inspired to participate in the Olympics because the reason that she had caught a later train that day was that she had been celebrating London being awarded the Olympic bid the night before. She had been faced with the need to deal with and adapt to a new way of being as someone with no legs, and choices about her future life.

Within that tragic injury, she glimpsed the potential of a different body.

One thing is certain in the journey through illness that we have been exploring in this series: human beings must deal with and adapt to change as they travel. This is a truism, of course, as we all have to deal with the changes brought about by age, but illness confronts us with change more abruptly than the more gradual alterations we may face as time passes. We have little choice but to accept the physical changes that illness brings, except in so far as we can choose or reject treatments or adaptations offered by medicine or other support services. Where we may have a choice, however, is in the kind of attitudes we adopt towards change. That choice can only be exercised if we are aware that we have options to adopt some attitudes or ways of being in relation to illness or disability, and not others. That requires awareness of the process of change: choosing to 'be' a certain way requires a sense of the process of 'becoming'.

In Volume three of this series, I made reference to the philosopher Havi Carel's discussion of adaptation to illness and its consequences in her book *Illness: the cry of the flesh.*[1] Carel refers to Heidegger's characterisation of human existence as 'being able to be': 'Human existence is characterised by its openness, potential, ability to become this or that thing.'[2] This is an attractive view of human life: that we have the power and freedom to shape our lives as we wish. But, as Carel points out, this power and freedom is not unlimited. The sense of bursting, burgeoning potential we may feel as young adults to be what we want to be is inevitably restricted as life progresses to old age by declining physical ability and capacity. For those dealing with the consequences of physical decline as a result of ill health, this sense of being restricted and having possibilities closed off can occur more suddenly, making loss of potential and choice stark and depressing.

The experience of 'inability' is, Carel argues, so common either as a result of illness or age, that Heidegger's definition of existence can be seen as excluding many people. She suggests two modifications:

> First the notion of 'being able to be' must be broadened to include radically differing abilities. Secondly, 'inability to be' needs to be recognized as a way of being. Heidegger's definition can be given an interesting twist if we think about being unable to be as a form of existence that is worthwhile, challenging and, most importantly, unavoidable. (p. 68.)

Martine Wright's inability led to new challenges and to a new way of being, but this was only possible because she recognised that her different body offered new potential. Her inability opened out new aspects of existence that were for her to choose or reject.

Doctors can get in the way of this kind of attitude towards the consequences of illness or disability because 'outcomes' often mark an end point in the medical process. Medicine is characteristically directed at treatment and at restoration; the effects of illness may be measured by the gap between previous abilities and current inability, making starker the reality of what has been lost. But the patient 'continues to be' beyond the consultation room and once treatment aimed at restoration has been exhausted. The patient may depart from medical intervention with a radically altered sense of how life may go on; he or she may be overwhelmed with a sense of inability or restricted possibility. The postscript to our patient Jake's story shows one way that life may go. For Jake, his life has been ruined by psoriasis: '[w]hat I really want is not to have had psoriasis.' This was not an option, but, except for his rejected girlfriend, Carol, no one encouraged him to think about what potential life had for him despite or even because of his condition. Rachel's rather dramatic story suggests that her sense of responsibility for the mix-up over Rachelle (that was not her fault) may awaken a dormant sense of responsibility for her own diabetes, and a forward trajectory of hope as she realises that her irresponsible attitude to her illness may have serious effects on others.

Acknowledging inability, having a sense of the possibilities of 'becoming' in other ways in life, can bring benefits in unexpected ways. Even the imminent approach of death can encapsulate a process of becoming that offers transcendence. As the political strategist Philip Gould wrote within days of his death on the day that he visited the site of his own grave:

> As this process goes on, as death gets closer, my experiences become more and more tense, but also more and more joyful. They are surprising too. Things happen that I would not have expected to happen. Coincidences occur. I find I have entered a world which is not how I thought it would be. It is much better than I thought it would be. The ground rules, the nature of reality, in this world, are different.[3]

This extract is full of Gould's astonishment at the joy he has found at the very end of his life. He expected to be full of sadness and regret, anticipating death at the relatively young age of 61 with a close, loving family and things he still wanted to do, while having to suffer from the unpleasant effects of oesophageal cancer. However, instead he is transcendent, amazed at the love and peace he has found in these final days.

What I want to explore, therefore, is the idea of 'becoming' in relation to what happens after and as a consequence of illness. As I have suggested, this concept emphasises the possibilities that emerge after illness rather than the potential that is closed down. It is more common to focus on the restrictions on ability and choice that occur in the context of reduced ability, but the fact that there is a process of becoming, between the existence before the illness and the being that results from it, suggests that there is a space and opportunity – that is ongoing – in which choice about the direction we take and the attitudes we adopt can affect outcomes. It may be that a greater awareness of this process and the power we may exercise over it may lie at the heart of a resilient response to illness.

BECOMING AND BEING: CHANGE, DISRUPTION AND CHOICE

Change

'Becoming' encapsulates a number of ideas. First, it is a process of change that leads from one thing to another. In this context, the process is from one way of being to another. But those two ways of being are not static points. 'Being' is dynamic and shifting and responsive to the world and the changing body.

If we think back on ourselves as children, it is sometimes difficult to imagine any sense of continuity between our 10-year-old self and our adult self. As the psychologist Nikolas Rose comments, '[Y]ou are more plural than you think.' He goes on to identify the philosophers Gilles Deleuze and Felix Guatarri as those who have articulated most radically an alternative view to the notion of subjectivity as 'coherent, enduring and individualised':

> You are a longitude and a latitude, a set of speeds and slownesses between unformed particles, a set of nonsubjectified affects. You have the individuality of a day, a season, a year, a *life* (regardless of its duration) – a climate, a wind, a fog, a swarm, a pack (regardless of its singularity).[4]

This is an exciting idea, radically expressed. We may look back on our 10-year-old selves with a sense of mystery, yet there are continuities. I remember my mother telling me at this age that I should not be too eager to please my friends and others. I recognise this to still be a trait of character that leads me into problems today! So there are continuities that are fundamental to who we are; aspects of character, preferences, skills, ways of relating to others and particular relationships that are the result of continuing love and commitment, make us uniquely ourselves. But to recognise that there is a dynamic aspect to being – that change occurs, adaptation takes place and we live on in a different way – can be reassuring and empowering.

Disruption

A second idea to consider about 'becoming' is that being is an embodied state, and that the process of becoming is also fully embodied; it is not just something that goes on in our heads. However, the body can at different times become more or less present in our sense of being. The changes brought about by illness tend to make the body more present in our conscious experience because it may be more difficult to do things that we could do before, like grasp a pen (for a patient with rheumatoid arthritis) or run for a bus (for a patient with chronic obstructive pulmonary disease (COPD)). Matthew Radcliffe writes about the idea of the 'conspicuous body':

> [W]hen involved in an activity, parts of the body can become immersed in that activity and often do not feature as objects of experience. Alternatively, they can become conspicuous, sometimes disrupting the activity in question. What we have is a range of different ways in which parts of the body can be felt, all of which are tied up with physical activity or withdrawal from it.[5]

Radcliffe, drawing on the philosophy of Martin Heidegger, describes the feeling of comfortable belonging to the world as being characterised by a familiarity with everyday objects and spaces that is determined by our habitual embodied interactions with them. Under these conditions, the body becomes less conspicuous, but it is nevertheless crucial to that sense of belonging:

> The body that falls into the background is not just the body that *acts*; it is the body that constitutes a sense of belonging, a context within which all purposive activities are embedded.[6]

When illness or disability affects our ability to interact with the familiar things of the world, the sense of belonging begins to disappear, and the body becomes more conspicuous as part of being. The historian and essayist Tony Judt, who died of amyotrophic lateral sclerosis (ALS) in 2012, wrote movingly of his unfamiliar feeling of utter focus on being in his body because of what that body could no longer do:

> With extraordinary effort I can move my right hand a little and can adduct my left arm some six inches across my chest. My legs, although they will lock when upright long enough to allow a nurse to transfer me from one chair to another, cannot bear my weight and only one of them has any autonomous movement left in it. … Having no use of my arms, I cannot scratch an itch, adjust my spectacles, remove food particles from my teeth or anything else which – as a moment's reflection will confirm – we all do dozens of times a day.[7]

In this extract, from his essay 'Night', the writing confirms the intense presence of the body in the forefront of Judt's experience because of the strangeness of being unable to 'scratch an itch' or carry out any of the, almost automatic, activities that 'we all do dozens of times a day'. The body here becomes conspicuous and leads to a change in the sense of belonging.[9]

One way of thinking about this is that through the process of 'becoming' – if we are to retain a sense of being at home in the world after illness – the body at first must become more conspicuous but then gradually recede as the changed body finds new ways of interacting with its environment. The success of this process may determine how patients flourish or otherwise in the changed circumstances in which they find themselves.

The implication here is that a disruption to the sense of belonging, which is signalled by the body coming to the fore and disrupting our automatic interactions with the world, is a negative thing to be overcome in the process of adapting to the outcomes of illness. However, as Carel stresses, the disruption that leads to adaptation does not necessarily need to be seen as negative. Adaptation is not just about 'coming to terms with illness or acceptance', both of which are passive responses.[10] Carel talks of adaptation taking place on a number of different levels: physical, but also psychological, social and temporal. Adaptation arises not as a response to a novel environment but as a response to changes in one's own body. Those of us who have been involved in foreign travel are familiar with the sense of disruption caused by being suddenly thrust into an unfamiliar environment and culture. This experience can increase physical awareness, and the body can feel out of place and clumsy in clothes that feel inappropriate or weather conditions that slow us down. But in dealing with the outcome of illness or disability, it is the strange body to which the patient must respond – a body that is unique to the patient and not shared by another. This adaptability is dependent upon resources that the patient has within herself or himself and that she or he draws from others. The responsive nature of adaptation also gives it what Carel terms a 'dialectic' nature, one of disruption followed by rapid response'. She goes on:

> The tension between the body as active and passive, subject and object, capable and unable, presented with an obstacle and overcoming it, is present in adaptability. It is not a smooth process but a series of dialectic encounters of a body with an environment, of a demand with failure, and of failure with the need for modification.[11]

This constant dialectic between the body and the environment, which leads to a response and adaptation, calls upon resources of imagination and creative thought that may not have been required when the body was in a kind of steady state with the environment – comfortable and at ease, belonging and in the background. Creativity is essential to adaptation, and may transform the experience of illness from one of negativity to one of positivity.

In her essay discussing the French writer Klossowski's book *Nietzsche and the Vicious Circle*, Eleanor Kaufman quotes a letter written by Nietzsche to his doctor. The cause of the suffering referred to in the letter was the severe migraines that came upon him without warning:

> My existence is a *dreadful burden*: I would have rejected it long ago, had I not been making the most instructive experiments in the intellectual and moral domain in just this condition of suffering and almost complete renunciation – this joyous mood, avid for knowledge, raised me to heights where I triumphed over every torture and all despair. On the whole, I am happier now than I have ever been in my life. And yet in continual pain; for many hours of the day, a sensation closely akin to seasickness, a semi- paralysis that makes it difficult to speak. … My only consolation is my thoughts and perspectives.[12]

Klossowski's interpretation of this passage is that for Nietzsche 'the act of thinking became identical with suffering, and suffering with thinking'. This is a strange idea, as for most of us the experience of pain is a distraction, focusing us on the body, making it difficult to think. But Klossowski here suggests that the physical excess experienced by Nietzsche in the form of his migraines 'allows for an unprecedented mental purity and freedom'.[13] Klossowski suggests that this occurs as a result of the disjunction between the body and the identity of the person:

> With respect to the sick body, the mind unleashes thought-energy that runs contrary to the negating forces of the body's sickness.[14]

Under these conditions, argues Kaufman, 'sickness or impurity is *not* a negative state to be overcome but rather a positive enabler that is never actually separate from its thought counterpart'.

In summary, then, the suggestion is that 'becoming' as an adaptation to illness involves disjunctions between the body and the mind. Those disjunctions are made apparent, for example, as the patient tries to fit an altered physical state into a familiar environment and experiences a dialectic between that unfamiliar state and the familiar world in which the mind and bodily responses oscillate between experiencing difficulty followed by problem solving to overcome it. This oscillation and trial and error is highly creative and releases what Kaufman terms 'thought sensations infused with corporeal energy'. Kaufman suggests that this represents the experience of a 'new cohesion':

> Provoked by the body, thought ascends to a space where it can revoke the body, but not without being energized by the body's very materiality.[15]

It may help here to turn to a couple of examples. Returning to Tony Judt's moving essay on his experience of the night, having been settled for sleep, his limbs set in positions to avoid bed sores and his glasses removed:

> [T]here I lie: trussed, myopic and motionless like a modern day mummy, alone in my corporeal prison, accompanied for the rest of the night only by my thoughts.[16]

His solution to what seems, for this active and gregarious man, an intolerable situation is to search among his thoughts, memories and fantasies for events that he can use 'to divert my mind from the body in which it is encased'. This is not easy, but he is 'occasionally astonished' at how this process enables him to rise above his physical circumstances. As he says: 'It's true that this disease has its enabling dimension: thanks to my inability to take notes or prepare them, my memory – already quite good – has improved considerably.' He is certainly not suggesting that he reaches a state of joy in his nightly wanderings, but this experience suggests that the idea of 'thought ascending to a space where it can revoke the body' can represent a becoming that allows a flourishing sense of being even under the circumstances of serious incurable illness.

Philip Gould's account of his experience of dying with oesophageal cancer also illustrates the nature of the dialectic between body, mind and environment that leads, in often imperceptible shifts, to adaptation and a new becoming. After his second serious operation at the Royal Victoria Infirmary (RVI) in Newcastle upon Tyne, he says that his worst moments were when the nurses changed his position in the bed:

> This always caused pain to shoot through my body like a small electric shock. With pain, as with almost everything else in cancer, the fear is worse than the reality, and every time you are able to defeat it your body and spirit become stronger. I still hate pain but I can now tolerate it in ways unimaginable three years ago.[17]

At this stage, he experiences the amazing ability of the body and human spirit to overcome difficulty and to change and become a person who is able to manage pain. The operation was not successful in curing his cancer and he suffered recurrence. Eventually he reached the stage where there was no hope at all that the cancer could be overcome, and he was told in no uncertain terms that he would be dead within six months. He and his wife responded to this news immediately by crying 'endlessly for hours'. Gould says that he 'was so sad.' This is an entirely appropriate response, but even this sadness, and the accompanying feeling that there was no escape, did not last even until the next day:

> A day later we bounced back. We just moved to a different place and a different time. It was a totally transcendent moment. I saw now that the purpose I had been seeking was to give as much love as I could. Even though I was dying I knew that was what I had to do. It was clear, there was absolutely no ambivalence about it. … And my life gained a kind of intensity that it had never had before. It gained a quality and a power that it had never had before.[18]

Like Nietzsche, Gould talks of being happier at this stage in his life than he ever was before,[19] and this passage explains the root of that happiness: that his being and its purpose have attained a clarity that he had never had before. The imminence of death has intensified the feeling of love he has for his family and friends, and this has become the pure object of his existence. This experience is entirely bound up with his embodied self. He describes a really rough night in which he was tired and sick for most of it. But through this he is supported by the presence of his wife, Gail. She is unable to do anything to assuage his physical distress but her attitude towards him provokes a transcendent response:

> I knew … that the tenderness I saw on her face was utterly dependent upon
> the knowledge that I was going to die, and that I would soon be dead. Without
> that knowledge of death there would have been no such tenderness, but with
> it, such tenderness was possible.[19]

In extremis, the pain and distress he feels in his body is translated into a feeling
of joy brought about by the response of another, which was, in its turn, only
possible because of that pain and distress. This dialectic moves Gould from a
position of despair and sadness to one of happiness and an accelerated sense of
becoming. He says within a few days of his death: 'I feel I am surging forward
and growing at a pace I have never experienced before' (p. 133).

In these two examples of people dealing with radical changes brought about
by illness, what is striking is the sense of astonishment both men experience at
their ability to find joy and release even under circumstances that most of us
would imagine to be intolerable. What I have suggested in this section is that
these unexpected and potentially positive responses are the result of the way in
which illness disrupts the smooth and unchallenging dialectic between the well
person and their environment. This disruption releases a creative response that
can enable people even in the most difficult circumstances of pain or situations
of inability to find new ways of being.

This is not, however, a universal experience. In August 2012, Tony
Nicklinson, who was paralysed from the neck down following a devastating
stroke, died a few days after being denied the legal right to support to end his
own life. Nicklinson described some of the same problems endured by Judt,
such as the fact that '90% of all itches have to be endured' because it takes
so long for him to explain where an itch is so that someone can scratch it
for him.[21] This he was able to put up with but what was intolerable for him,
and for some others in a similar position, was the fact that if life became too
much to bear, he had no way out. He was unable to choose not to be. The
problem, and what made life impossible for him (and for people like Debbie
Purdey who suffers from multiple sclerosis (MS)), was not the effects of the
illness itself, but rather the way in which it denied him the right to make
fundamental choices, such as whether to live or die.

Choice and becoming

Nicklinson was adapting in some ways to his illness (he could tolerate
itches) but his capacity to continue with life was hampered by his lack
of choice. There seemed to be no sense from his experience of becoming a
patient with locked-in syndrome in which that process of becoming had, like
for Judt or Gould, released options for ways of being – like a new series of
unexpected doors opening on lives unimagined before illness. What then
makes it possible for some people to deal with the outcomes of illness better

than others? What influences becoming, and how is it possible to arrive at a situation where those new doors open rather than at a feeling that as old doors close, there is nothing else?

As a way into thinking about this and the important role choice – or lack of it – may play, it may be useful to examine what resources an understanding of the process of becoming reveals. So far, I have described 'becoming' as being characterised by change over time. This lends us insight. We know that development is possible: that we are able to be a different person in a changed body because we can look back on our childhood selves seeing continuities but also transformation. I have also stressed the embodied nature of becoming and how the necessary responses we have to make to the changes in our bodies after illness in the context of familiar environments can lead to the release of creative energy. These two characteristics of 'becoming' enable choice. Time gives the patient opportunities to examine options, to learn what works and what does not and to adopt different approaches to the consequence of illness. The release of creative energy allows for a sense of potential and the generation of possibilities.

What I have described here, however, relates to an idea of the self that is *intra*subjective rather than *inter*subjective. The kind of dialectic that is part of becoming does not just involve interactions between self (body and mind) and the physical world, it involves exchanges with the attitudes and beliefs of others in domestic and work spaces, with societal values and ways of thinking, with cultural norms and projected values of beauty and appropriateness and also with the categories and structures of medical practice. These attitudes, structures and norms are often rather rigid and unresponsive to the dialectic of individual becoming and may, in consequence, get in the way of creativity and change.

One example of how such structures can interfere with the process of becoming is in the sphere of public health. Women who smoke in pregnancy have been the subject of study because of the potential for problems such as low birth-weight and effects on the continuing health of the baby and child. The outcome for individual pregnant women smokers is highly dependent on their social status. Women who come from more advantaged backgrounds are less likely to smoke in the first place, are more likely to succeed in quitting while pregnant and are more likely to remain non-smokers.[22] What these disadvantaged women smokers experience during pregnancy is the full force of medical and societal disapproval. They report feelings of guilt and low self-worth, and many seem caught in a constant confusing carousel of attempting to give up, struggling to sustain a quit attempt and lapsing back with relief but with continued feelings of guilt fuelled by public health advice and the disapproval of their partners, who are often smokers themselves.[23] From a public health perspective, the 'becoming' trajectory of a pregnant smoker is clearly normative: give up or you risk damaging your baby. For the woman herself, smoking may be the only thing that supports her through a complex and difficult life dealing with a toddler, with problems relating to housing and finances and disrupted social networks that result from giving up work. Individual women in this situation may suffer from a confusion of influences on their becoming as smokers or non-smokers. They may enjoy smoking and may find relief and relaxation from it, but they do not perceive that they are free to make choices about smoking or not, or about finding a level that may mean cutting down to those few essential cigarettes that support their 'being' in pregnancy, but which also confer least risk on their child. The rigid 'you must quit' of public health advice reduces the kind of becoming that they may naturally achieve.[24]

It is very difficult, as a patient with a chronic illness dependent on advice and support from your doctor, or as a vulnerable single mother struggling through a pregnancy with other young children, to break free from the confines of medical prognosis about what you will be or should do: to exercise choice in becoming. The freedom to become in unexpected ways may be obstructed by the weight of expectation: that because people are 'selves of a particular type'[25] with illnesses and disabilities of a particular type, they will behave and respond in ways predicted by biomedical or epidemiological research. Havi Carel suggests that medical practitioners may have a role in supporting openness in adaptation and freedom in becoming:

> I believe that medical practitioners would do well to adopt a broader, less exclusively naturalistic approach if they want to assist their chronically ill patients maintain [or extend] their habits, activities and goals. The naturalistic approach provides only a limited, biological picture of illness and therefore fails to help us understand the experience of illness.[26]

'LET US NOT WASTE OUR TIME GRIZZLING': FLOURISHING IN BECOMING

At the beginning of this chapter, I wrote of Martine Wright, who overcame the terrible loss of both of her legs to become a Paralympic athlete. Finding herself lying in bed in hospital after the 7/7 bombings she looked down at the blanket and discovered that her legs were not there:

> That's when I realized I had a choice – I could either lie down and never walk again, or I could get up and carry on with life, whatever the future might hold.[27]

Her remarkable becoming, from a person whose body was ravaged by bombs to Olympic athlete, exemplifies a number of the features that support flourishing within illness and disability. 'Becoming' in response to chronic illness and disability happens whatever the patient does, but 'successful' becoming, or becoming that leads to happiness within illness or disability is dependent first and foremost on awareness that change will happen, is inevitable and is part of life. Awareness of the forward movement of becoming allows the patient the capacity to choose what attitudes or aims they may adopt in response to the dialectic set up between their changed body and the physical world and relational environment in which they live. Wright realised she had a choice and decided on the course that she would follow. Diana Athill, writing at the age of 89 regarding the decline of old age, exhibits a similar enabling awareness:

> We [old people] tend to become convinced that everything is getting worse simply because within our own boundaries things *are* doing so. We are becoming less able to do things we would like to do, can hear less, eat less, hurt more, our friends die, we know that we ourselves will soon be dead. ... It's not surprising, perhaps, that we easily slide into a general pessimism about life. ... Whereas if, flitting in and out of our awareness, there are people who are beginning, to whom the years ahead are long and full of who knows what, it is a reminder – indeed it enables us actually to feel again – that we are not just dots at the end of thin black lines projecting into nothingness, but are parts of the broad, many-coloured river teeming with beginnings, ripenings, decayings, new beginnings – are still parts of it, and our dying will be part of it just as these children's being young is, so while we still have the equipment to see this, let us not waste our time grizzling.[28]

I quoted this wonderful passage from Athill's book *Somewhere Towards the End* in full because not only does it demonstrate the value of awareness, but also the importance of the second feature of successful becoming, that of adaptability, which requires openness and flexibility. If in the course of the disruption experienced as a result of our changed sense of embodiment we are continually seeking restoration to the way that things were before, we are likely to be frustrated and disappointed. Jake cannot have 'life without psoriasis' and Liz's chances of having another child may be slim. There is no turning back the clock.

Choices are open to those who feel themselves to have an internal locus of control.[29] But it is more likely that patients will develop this sense of agency if medical and health practitioners are themselves aware of the larger hinterland of life and opportunity that is not wholly determined by considerations of health and ability. 'Being unable to be' what the patient was before illness is the starting point for a new process of becoming. Accepting that and being aware of one's own choices and power to construct a new becoming may be the start of flourishing 'being' in the face of illness outcomes.

REFERENCES

1. Carel H. *Illness: the cry of the flesh*. Stocksfield: Acumen; 2008.
2. Ibid. p. 66.
3. Gould P. *When I Die: lessons from the death zone*. London: Little, Brown; 2012. p. 139.
4. Rose N. *Inventing Ourselves: psychology, power and personhood*. Cambridge: Cambridge University Press; 1996. p. 170. Emphasis in original.
5. Deleuze and Guatarri quoted in Rose N. op. cit. p. 170.
6. Radcliffe M. *Feelings of Being: phenomenology, psychiatry and the sense of reality*. Oxford: Oxford University Press; 2008. p. 112. Emphasis in original.
7. Ibid. p. 112.
8. Judt T. Night. *New York Review of Books*. 57(1). 14 January 2010.
9. Radcliffe M. op. cit. p. 112.
10. Carel H. op. cit. p. 81.
11. Ibid.
12. Kaufman E. 'Klossowski or thoughts-becoming'. In: Grosz E, editor. *Becomings: explorations in time, memory and futures*. New York, NY: Cornell University Press; 1999. pp. 141–57. Emphasis in original.
13. Ibid. p. 153.
14. Ibid.
15. Ibid. p. 154. Emphasis in original.
16. Judt T. op. cit.
17. Gould P. op. cit. p. 73.
18. Ibid. p. 125.
19. Ibid. p. 129.
20. Ibid. p. 128.
21. BBC News. *Assisted Dying Debate: Tony Nicklinson in his own words*. Available at: www.bbc.co.uk/news/uk-england-wiltshire-18398797 (accessed 19 October 2012).
22. Graham H., Sowden A, Flemming K, *et al*. *Using Qualitative Research To Inform Interventions To Reduce Smoking In Pregnancy In England: a systematic review of qualitative studies*. Public Health Research Consortium Short Report, October 2011.
23. Ibid.
24. Macnaughton J, Carro-Ripalda S, Russell A. 'Risking enchantment': how are we to view the smoking person? *Critical Public Health*. 2012; **22**(6): 455–69.
25. Rose N. op. cit. p. 169.
26. Carel H. op. cit. p. 87.
27. Martine Wright quoted in 'From 7/7 victim to Paralympic inspiration: sitting volleyball captain Martine Wright's incredible journey'. *The Mirror* online. 28 August 2012. Available at: www.mirror.co.uk/sport/other-sports/paralympics-2012-martine-wright---1283933 (accessed 21 October 2012).
28. Athill D. *Somewhere Towards the End*. London: Granta; 2009. p. 84. Emphasis in original.
29. Richardson GE. The metatheory of resilience and resilience. *Journal of Clinical Psychology*. 2002; **58**: 307–21.

7

Prognosis or prophecy?

JILL GORDON

A woman whose husband had advanced prostate cancer came to see me. She mentioned, in the course of the consultation, that she was afraid that her husband was being 'ripped off' by a charlatan. He had exhausted conventional treatments and was now paying a lot of money for a special cancer medicine that was being sent to him in the post. Did I think that sounded right? She had expressed her concern to her husband, but he had become quite angry and said that she was only objecting to the treatment because of the cost. 'You're worried that I'll spend all our money before I die.' That was, in truth, a key concern, assuming that the 'special medicine' was indeed a scam.

I asked whether she and her husband would like me to look into it any further. A few days later she made an appointment for both of them to see me. In that consultation, her husband, Dr P, told me that he too wanted to know whether he could trust his therapist. He had asked the prostate specialist what he thought about it and the specialist had told him that the alternative treatment would probably do no harm. (I gritted my teeth. How do you know it cannot do harm if you do not know what is in it?)

I asked Dr P if he would like me to go ahead to find out more, and he said 'yes'. His wife smiled.

Meanwhile, I suggested that he himself may like to find out more about the therapist's qualifications. Since Dr P was a retired physicist, he had an idea of the kind of university degree or other qualification he may expect his therapist to hold. On being asked, however, the 'therapist' sent back a scathing email that said, in part, that if he did not have Dr P's full trust he would prefer not to continue the treatment. He did not offer any evidence of qualifications.

As for me, it didn't take much searching to find a newspaper article that I still have on file. The article provided evidence of the man's interesting criminal record including a period of time in jail for a bank robbery. I called the reporter who had written the article and found that this man had been investigated on many occasions for making false claims about his power to heal. He had even set up his own 'clinic' for fellow prisoners!

In addition to purporting to cure cancer he was supplying receipts for Dr P to submit to his private health insurer for reimbursement of face-to-face consultations. The consultations had in fact been much fewer in number and all but the first one were by telephone.

Finally Dr and Mrs P returned to ask what I had found out. I laid out the newspaper articles, with stories of other 'patients' who had trusted his cures and later found out that they had been deceived. He had no qualifications at all. I told them about the reporter who had written the exposé. The woman sat wide-eyed, reading the articles. Staring hard at me, Dr P said only, 'You have just robbed me of my last hope.'

A few months later, he died.

HOPE

'You have just robbed me of my last hope.'

Surely that can't be true.

I give, rather than take; I give expert help to people in need – diagnosis and treatment. I give guidance; I give support; I give hope. People are rightly grateful.

How could I have 'robbed' Dr P?

Did I make a misjudgement?

Was there no choice but the choice between harsh truth and false hope?

My motives seemed clear to me at the time. First, I felt sympathy for the woman whose respect for her husband was slipping away as she observed his inability to face his death calmly and with honesty and dignity. I also felt repelled by the idea that anyone would use manipulation and threats to extort money from a dying man. Finally, I was confident that, as a man of science, Dr P would thank me for helping to illuminate the path towards truth.

In my ideal scenario, Dr P would have recognised what Robert Frost observed just before his death: 'In three words I can sum up everything I've learned about life — it goes on.' For me, those simple words reflect a broadening of perspective, an acceptance of the continuity of life in which each individual participates for just a short period of time. His words say, in effect, I am not the centre of the universe.

I had hoped that an accurate prognosis may help Dr P to make use of the time remaining to him for any necessary reconciliation and for a last affirmation of love and pride and gratitude to family and friends. An accurate prognosis may clear a way to a dignified and calm death, grounded in the knowledge that, as Socrates pointed out, there is little to fear, and indeed

> there is great reason to hope that death is a good, for one of two things: either death is a state of nothingness and utter unconsciousness, or, as men say, there is a change and migration of the soul from this world to another [where] I shall be able to continue my search into true and false knowledge; as in this world, so also in that; I shall find out who is wise and who pretends to be wise.

As a scientist, Dr P had been steeped in that 'search for true and false knowledge' and it was hard to understand how he could have been duped, when there were so many warning signs, and his own wife had expressed such misgivings. It had been quite easy for me to find out that his 'saviour' was actually a criminal; surely he himself could have done the same?

But perhaps I was too keen to declare the triumph of science over what I had perceived as ingenuousness. My frustration grew in proportion with my certainty, a dangerous state of mind. What an irony that I was so certain that he should be more uncertain about his 'saviour'!

From Dr P's perspective, he knew only too well that scientists do not know everything. He had been effectively abandoned by the cancer specialist who told him that the alternative treatments 'could do no harm.' Meanwhile he suspected that his wife was more concerned about the cost of the alternative treatment than its potential benefits, and finally, he had only a reluctant relationship with me, initiated by his wife, rather than a trusting relationship based on his own perceived need. In Chapter 4 Carl Edvard Rudebeck writes about the primacy of the commitment between doctor and patient, even before they meet, which is a key implication of Levinas's position that ethics constitutes 'first philosophy', ahead of questions of ontology and epistemology.

This commitment receives scant attention in medical school and among healthcare providers. Medical diagnosis, treatment and prognosis all depend on our ability to manipulate complex data in a 'thinking space' where there are no patients, but merely facts.[1,2] It is a struggle to keep the commitment at the heart of day-to-day practice, but we know intuitively that something is missing when this commitment is lost. The profession's ambivalent response to the evidence-based medicine movement may be partly explained by a fear that abstracted information about groups of patients will trump clinical judgement and intuition concerning the care of individuals.[3,4] In Volume 2, John Saunders reflected on the contribution that personal judgement makes in the process of diagnosis, in its blending of rationality and intuition:

> In scientific discovery, personal judgement is brought to bear in a way that cannot be described even in principle. There is an element of connoisseurship in arriving at such judgments, just as there is in identifying (diagnosing?) a fine wine, portraying a Shakespearian character or making a Stradivarius violin. The roots for such knowing may be mainly tacit and no computer could replace them. (p 150)

It is this embodied world of space and time that provides the relational elements that purely medical/technical thinking strips away. In Volume 1 Carl Edvard Rudebeck explored the experience of the lived body as 'existential anatomy' – the body in space – and in Chapter 4 of this volume he explores the centrality of time to the moral commitment created in the doctor–patient relationship, an element that was partly missing in my relationship with Dr P.

The fact that we apprehend the world and one another in essentially different ways may help to explain the tension that led to my moral dilemma. On the one hand, an understanding of medical science, an understanding of cancer treatment (and an understanding of the fact that there will always be scammers who prey on vulnerable people) – all of the rational elements that make up my worldview – seemed to impose a moral imperative to save Dr P from his own foolishness. On the other hand, his own unique experience of himself and his relationship to the world and his recourse to magical thinking were what was holding him during this time of crisis. The challenge that I faced and failed was to fully understand these things; the fake medicine was making Dr P feel better, but the mechanism for the benefit was not to be found in science, which had become his enemy. His only friend was hope, and a false hope prevailed over a true prognosis.

Some Australian researchers have studied the phenomenon of hope among patients with cancer and the doctors and nurses who look after them.[5] In examining the way they talk about cancer, the researchers found that people tend to think of Hope (the noun) as an aspect of the official prognosis. To say, 'There is no Hope,' means that treatment has, officially, failed; care from now on will be palliative. But this does not mean that the patient, the family, the doctors and the nurses will not go on hoping – and hoping – and hoping. In this latter sense, hope – as a verb rather than a noun – is an irrepressible activity. It can be an active, courageous refusal to be silenced by illness. It can be a reaching out toward the least possibility of a future, however slim the hope may be.

As Martyn Evans points out in the last chapter, we have no way of experiencing a state of non-being. Our metaphors about death are necessarily material in nature: death as parting or as sleep, the end of a story or the beginning of a new 'chapter'. It is not possible to reverse Descartes's 'cogito, ergo sum' and say 'non sum, ergo non cogito'. The self-contradictory nature of the task reminds us that we are always thinking, one way or another, about the things that are and the things that are not. From those things that are, we create those things that are not – the products of the imagination. These are an amalgam of 'real' things – the world of unicorns and angels. So when we try to think about death, imagination moves in the only direction that it can: if death is inevitable, then life must be transformed into 'after-life'. And if an afterlife is possible, may not other miracles be possible, too – a miracle cure, perhaps?

I suspect that Dr P could not escape the realisation that the promise of a cure was false. Perhaps his anger was in proportion to that repressed scepticism. His wife wanted him to be realistic – to talk to his adult children about his prognosis and to make arrangements for the last stage of his life. He wanted to remain in a space where his imagination may yet defy the remorseless march of the disease. Who can say who was right?

PROGNOSIS

Dr P's story illustrates the tensions between scientific medicine and the traditions of non-scientific medical healing. Both are vulnerable to exploitation, and while most of our attention in this *Companion* series has been focused on a critique of scientific medicine without the mediating hand of healing, the 'hand of healing' without the mediating hand of science is potentially harmful, too. At the very least it leads to the waste of an enormous amount of money that could be used to support medical care that actually works.

The power of science lies in its capacity for prognostication, and prognosis is not to be confused with prophecy. Weather forecasters illustrate the point. They are wrongly maligned for being mere prognosticators and not prophets. The same can be said of the experts in global warming or financial trends or terrorism. In each example, the experts make prognoses; that is, they use past experience and their expert judgement to predict the likely future behaviour of the planet's ecosystem, the movement of capital or the behaviour of psychopathic ideologues. It is sometimes difficult to remember that prognoses are subject to all sorts of intervening effects that may change the actual outcome; prognoses are not prophecies.

Following the 2009 L'Aquila, Italy, earthquake that killed 309 people, a court in Italy sentenced seven scientists to six years in jail for manslaughter. The men were found guilty of failing to adequately warn the public about the imminent risk of a major earthquake. The indictment accused them of giving 'inexact, incomplete and contradictory information'. The prosecutors argued that deaths in the earthquake could have been avoided had people not been reassured by one of the experts that the situation was 'normal'. There was clearly confusion in people's minds about what constitutes a 'normal' situation in L'Aquila. 'Normal' implied 'safe' to the people of the town, but, for the scientists, 'normal' meant no change in risk, and for the judges 'normal' was inexact and incomplete.

But how do we agree on a definition of what is normal and abnormal in an area prone to earthquakes? Scientists are able to make long-term projections about the likelihood of earthquakes, but short-term predictions (within days or hours) are simply not possible.[7] If the threshold for warning the residents is sufficiently low, notifications in areas like Christchurch, San Francisco or Tokyo would need to be sounded on a continual basis.

As with earthquakes, a medical prognosis is merely a forecast based on the best evidence available at that time. It makes estimates about the possible outcomes of illness using data from other people who are alike in key ways, such as, age, sex and ethnicity. It literally gathers up those data to create a distribution curve, which is commonly 'normal' in shape. It allows us to say that 'people with this condition normally recover completely' or 'people with this condition normally die within five years.'

When a prognosis is made, it is quickly converted to a prophecy by both patients and their families. 'They said he'd be dead in six months, and here it is, ten months later and he is still alive. The doctors were wrong.' Once a number or period is spoken – 'perhaps six months', 'possibly a year' – the 'perhaps' and the 'possibly' are soon stripped away. But prognosis is simply a statement of likely outcomes. There is no mystique in prognostication. For the doctor sitting face to face with Rachel, Jake, Liz, Geoff or Jen, the art of care lies in taking valid data from the history, investigations and examination, and combining them with what is known about a particular type of illness. The decisions that are made about the care of individual patients are necessarily based on what we know about the natural history of disease and the benefit, or lack of benefit, from a medical intervention to render the natural history 'unnatural' through effective treatment. Prognoses are a cornerstone of healthcare – without them we could not justify the pain and the indignity experienced by Rachel, Jake, Liz, Geoff and Jen in the course of their respective treatments.

When we first met Rachel in Volume 1, she was a little girl newly diagnosed with diabetes. Past experience enables us to make a prognosis regarding what would have happened to her without treatment – this condition was once fatal. Her 'unnatural' prognosis, thanks to the discovery of insulin, is to live an almost normal life, provided that she sticks to her treatment plan and a sensible lifestyle. But the very insulin that is lifesaving for Rachel is life-threatening for Rachelle, the young woman who happened to be in the same hospital room when Rachel was admitted with hyperglycaemia. Who could have predicted that Rachel's brief absence from her bed could have allowed a mix-up to occur with such a devastating outcome, and who could possibly hold her responsible? The answer of course, is Rachel herself: 'If only I'd stayed put. If only I'd been there when the nurse came to give me that insulin. It's all my fault.'

Rachel's reaction is typical of the way that we all think. Whether we realise it or not, superstition is rife. How often do you hear: 'When your number's up, your number's up'. Or 'Everything happens for a reason'. Scientific thinking is not 'natural' to human minds; we would much prefer to take a variety of shortcuts – shortcuts that have served us more or less well in the past. We seek out a guru, flip a coin, rely on magic or construct a belief system that will tell us what to do. In the wake of the Second World War Erich Fromm observed humankind to be suffering from 'the fear of freedom'[10] and Doris Lessing identified the way our minds construct what she called 'prisons we choose to live inside'.[11] Both of them drew attention to the difficulties posed by living with uncertainty, and our preference for false certainty. Bertrand Russell put it even more succinctly when he said that '*most people would rather die than think. In fact, they often do*'.

But certainty is dangerous, even while it is comforting. The charlatan who treated Dr P claimed special knowledge of how cancer 'works', and how to beat it. There are always people willing to offer magic cures, whether they are for Rachel's diabetes, Jake's psoriasis, Liz's and Jen's cancer or Geoff's dementia. They are like the crocodile in Alice's Adventures in Wonderland:

> How cheerfully he seems to grin,
> How neatly spread his claws,
> And welcomes little fishes in,
> With gently smiling jaws.

If a rational scientist like Dr P can fall victim to false hope, what chance does the uneducated person have of finding his or her way around the maze of medical jargon? Medical specialisation is now so great that doctors themselves cannot understand colleagues in other specialties, far less keep up to date with advances in all fields of medicine. What is more, some health professionals are willing to exploit people's difficulty in perceiving the difference between prognosis and prophecy. Book stores are full of promises for 'medically proven' weight loss programmes written by doctors who are willing to pit themselves against orthodox medicine. When challenged they make claims to knowledge beyond 'mere science'.

In Volume 3 of our *Companion* series, Rolf Ahlzén described how the German physician Franz Mesmer 'mesmerised' a gullible public into accepting his theory of animal magnetism. Harriet Hall,[12] a family physician who writes on scientific thinking in medicine, provides a neat summary of the characteristics of the medical prophet. She tells us how to recognise the 'lone genius', as represented by Mesmer *et al.* The story usually follows along these lines:

1. witnesses an unexpected improvement after a treatment
2. assumes that the treatment caused the improvement

3. does not test this assumption or try to rule out other possible explanations
4. proceeds to treat many other patients the same way, with apparent success, and allows confirmation bias to bolster his or her conviction
5. ego is boosted by grateful patients and by the conviction that he or she has special knowledge
6. extends the treatment to patients with other diagnoses
7. exercises his or her imagination and speculates about a possible physiological mechanism by which the treatment may work
8. generalises, often claiming to have found the 'one cause of all disease'
9. tries to convince scientists by describing his or her anecdotal experiences
10. scientists refuse to accept his or her untenable explanations or to publish his or her scientifically unacceptable papers
11. accuses the scientific establishment of persecuting him or her and suppressing knowledge that would undermine the status quo and help many patients
12. plays the lone genius card, often comparing himself to Galileo or Semmelweis
13. writes books and sells things.

Dr Hall draws our attention to a host of Mesmer's successors. Dr Fereydoon Batmanghelidj[12] contended that dehydration is the root of all evil. DD Palmer[13] invented chiropractic after convincing himself that a back adjustment restored a deaf janitor's hearing. Samuel Hahnemann[14] experienced malaria-like symptoms after taking an anti-malarial, thus stimulating his homeopathic theory. Edward Bach[15] based his Bach Flower Remedies on his intuitive psychic connection with various plants. Francine Shapiro[16] invented 'eye movement desensitisation and reprocessing' (EMDR) after noticing that feelings of anxiety were reduced when she looked around her during a walk in the park.[17] The similarities with mesmerism are obvious, but proponents of EMDR have cleverly manipulated the tenets of evidence based medicine (EBM) to create a huge amount of 'evidence' for its benefits, demonstrating that it is possible to subvert even the best of intentions and to turn a simple relaxation technique into a lucrative industry.

PROPHECY

The Ancient Greek *prohemi* simply means 'to foretell'. *Prediction*, from the Latin, is similar in meaning, if not quite as strong in tone. It means literally 'saying beforehand'. We tend to talk about prophecy when we think about myths and legends, while we talk about prediction when we think in cooler, more scientific terms, of the weather or the results of the next election. Prophecy is central to religious belief and is often a key component of myths and legends.

In either case, the prophet is often a creature from another world, a strange old man, a fairy or a witch. Within religious context, prophets usually promise reward for upright behaviour and threaten punishment for bad. In many cases prophets communicate across the divide between the immaterial and the material world. Being selected for this task can be a curse; think of Cassandra and her foreknowledge that Troy must inevitably fall.

Dark prophecies are found in tragedies from Sophocles's *Oedipus Rex* to Shakespeare's *Macbeth* and *Lear*. We understand exactly what is meant by the phrases 'Greek tragedy' and 'self-fulfilling prophecy'. In fairy stories, the prophecy has a lighter touch; Fate is not the remorseless monster that destroys all in its path. We look forward to the clever twist that ensures the triumph of good over evil. In *The Sleeping Beauty* a baby princess is cursed by an evil fairy at her christening ceremony. The fairy makes the prophecy that she will prick her finger on a spinning wheel and die. Despite a royal order to remove all of the spinning wheels from the castle, we are not surprised when the curious princess finds a spindle and pricks her finger. Does she die? Of course not – a good fairy has already prophesied that she will merely sleep for 100 years, and be woken by a handsome prince. So it is that we comfort our children and ourselves. Fairy stories have many such imbedded values. In recent times the *Harry Potter* stories have been attacked for their 'anti-Christian' values[8] and contrasts drawn with CS Lewis's Narnia where good and evil, conflict and redemption are refracted through the lens of the Christian belief system.[9]

Whether in Greek tragedies, in Shakespeare or in fairy tales, the gift of prophecy has the power to suspend natural law and thereby change the future. In the modern world, powerful medical treatments almost achieve that end in modifying the natural history of a disease. At times it seems that prognosis comes very close to prophecy.

SUPERSTITION

You've broken a mirror? Seven years bad luck. You've blown out all of the candles on your birthday cake? Your wish will be granted. A superstition is, according to the *Merriam-Webster* online dictionary, 'a belief or practice resulting from ignorance, fear of the unknown, trust in magic or chance, or a false conception of causation'. As irrational as superstitious behaviour may appear, evolutionary biologists are coming around to the idea that superstitious behaviour may actually have had survival advantages.[18] Foster and Kokko have shown that superstitious behaviours may have been rewarded in the process of natural selection. They point out that natural selection accommodates strategies that lead to frequent errors as long as the occasional correct response carries a large survival benefit. Because survival depends on so many different factors, there may be conditions under which natural selection can favour associated events that are never causally related. Behaviours that are, or appear to be, superstitious, are therefore inevitable.

Why it matters

The belief systems that lie behind prognosis and prophecy represent radically different worldviews. Prognoses are guarded and contingent on other events. Prophecies are never wrong; Shakespeare went to great lengths to ensure that the witches' prophecies in *Macbeth* were fulfilled, even if the reasoning was outrageously questionable.

Prophecy is much more exciting than prognosis, and it is tempting to believe that it is harmless. A benign prophecy simply puts a positive spin on future prospects. In times past doctors were even encouraged to construct benign prophecies in order to 'spare' patients from the truth. Surely that's not unreasonable.

It's certainly in line with everyday thinking. 'Whatever will be, will be,' expresses a fatalistic belief that our futures are foreordained. Whenever a patient expresses the belief that 'everything happens for the best', a rational response may be to say: 'No; not everything happens for the best. Tyrants, illnesses, accidents, and natural disasters don't happen for the best. Humans may have the capacity to see the best hidden somewhere in the debris of our lives, but disasters don't happen in order to give us the opportunity to pick through the rubble to find consolation for the misery they cause.'

The idea of an honest prognosis reminds me of a story by Irvin Yalom about a man whose true prognosis was of inestimable value in changing his life course. In the story 'If Rape were Legal',[19] Yalom describes 'Carlos' who had exploited others throughout his life, including his own children. His experience of psychotherapy following a brutally honest prognosis helps him to turn the remainder of his life around. Yalom was his treating psychiatrist and the story closes with these words:

> In the few months of life remained to him, Carlos … was a marvelously gener-
> ous and supportive father. … He gave no greater gift than the one he offered
> me shortly before he died, and it was a gift that answers for all time the ques-
> tion of whether it is rational or appropriate to strive for 'ambitious' therapy
> in those who are terminally ill. When I visited him in the hospital he was so
> weak he could barely move, but he raised his head, squeezed my hand and
> whispered, 'Thank you. Thank you for saving my life.' (p86)

Carlos's transformation did not come from any dissimulation about a benign prognosis with respect to his cancer. Instead he becomes aware of a much more odious prognosis, if his careless wish for rape to be legal were ever fulfilled. In therapy he gradually becomes aware of the significance of Kant's categorical imperative that we act only according to a maxim that we would be willing to accept as a universal law.

The relationship that Carlos developed with Yalom helped him to appreciate that facing his grim prognosis might help him to change his life and his relationships: 'His death was not one of the dark, muffled, conspiratorial passings. Until the very end of his life, he and his children were honest with one another about his illness and giggled together at the way he snorted, crossed his eyes, and puckered his lips when he referred to his "lymphoooooooooooomma".' (p86)

If it is difficult to find a truly benign form of prophecy in medicine, may it be possible to identify a malign form of prognosis? Dr P would almost certainly have said that I was guilty of delivering one, but the truth must surely be found in the intention. The prognosis, by itself, is value neutral – it is the end result of a process of data gathering, analysis and synthesis.

A prognosis can only be malign in delivery and application, rather than in content – presented perhaps in the form of a punishment. Today's 'lifestyle diseases' present great scope for guilt and a sense of failure,[20] as Pekka Louhiala outlines in the chapter that follows.

When Jane visits the grave of her sister Jen, in our final story, she asks herself: 'Life. Where does it take us? What does it all mean? What is it for?' These age-old questions have explanations that are, as HL Mencken put it, 'neat, plausible, and wrong'. How tempting it is for doctors to take on the role of prophet and sage, rather than adapting and responding to the uniqueness of each experience of illness.

REFERENCES

1. Groopman J. *How Doctors Think*. Boston, MA: Houghton Mifflin; 2007.
2. McGilchrist I. *The Master and His Emissary: the divided brain and the making of the Western world*. New Haven, CT: Yale Universty Press; 2009.
3. Downie RS and Macnaughton J. *Clinical Judgement: evidence in practice*. Oxford: Oxford University Press; 200.
4. Barratt A. Evidence based medicine and shared decision making: the challenge of getting both evidence and preferences into health care. Patient Education and Counselling. 2008; **73**: 407–12.
5. Eliott J and Olver I. Hope and hoping in the talk of dying cancer patients. *Social Science & Medicine*. 2007; **64**: 138–49.
6. Fingarette H. *Death: philosophical soundings*. Open Court Publishing; 1996.
7. Pritchard C. L'Aquila ruling: should scientists stop giving advice? *BBC News Magazine*. London: BBC; 2012.
8. Abanes R. *Harry Potter and the Bible: the menace behind the magick*. Camp Hill, PA: Horizon; 2001.
9. Caughey S, editor. *Revisiting Narnia: fantasy, myth and religion in CS Lewis's chronicles*. Dallas, TX: BenBella Books; 2005.

10. Fromm E. *The Fear of Freedom*. London: Routledge and Kegan Paul; 1942.
11. Lessing D. *Prisons We Choose To Live Inside*. Concord, Canada: Anansi; 1987.
12. Siminoff LA, Graham GC, Gordon NH. Cancer communication patterns and the influence of patient characteristics: disparities in information-giving and affective behaviors. *Patient Education and Counseling*. 2006; **62**(3): 355–60.
13. Palmer D. *The Science, Art and Philosophy of Chiropractic*. Portland, OR: Portland Printing House Company; 1910.
14. Hahnemann S. *The Chronic Diseases, Their Specific Nature and Their Homeopathic Treatment: antipsoric remedies*. Hempel CJ, editor. Michigan: Scholarly Publishing Office, University of Michigan; 1845.
15. Bach E. *The Essential Writings Of Dr Edward Bach: the twelve healers and heal thyself*. London: Random House; 2005.
16. Shapiro F. *Eye Movement Desensitization and Reprocessing: basic principles, protocols, and procedures*. New York, NY: Guildford Press; 2001.
17. McNally RJ. EMDR and mesmerism: a comparative historical analysis. *Journal Of Anxiety Disorders*. 1999; **13**(1–2): 225–36.
18. Foster KR and Kokko H. The evolution of superstitious and superstition-like behaviour. *Proceedings of the Royal Society B: biological sciences*. 2009; **276**(1654): 31–7.
19. Yalom I. *Love's Executioner and Other Tales Of Psychotherapy*. New York, NY: Harper Perennial; 1990.
20. Marlow LAV, Waller J, Wardle J. Variation in blame attributions across different cancer types. *Cancer Epidemiology Biomarkers & Prevention*. 2010; **19**(7): 1799–1805.

8

First do no harm

PEKKA LOUHIALA

The medical establishment has become a major threat to health.[1]

[S]ince biomedical research saves lives, it is unsurprising that the regulation of research costs lives.[2]

The pendulum has swung from rather crass paternalism practised fifty or sixty years ago to an obsession with autonomy which allows patients with questionable autonomy to come to harm.[3]

One of modern medicine's outcomes is its potential to do harm. If there are medical effects, there may be side effects. The types of harm that the practice of medicine can cause are many. They are sometimes intended, like the short-term harm necessarily caused in surgical operations. They are sometimes unintended but predictable, as with common side effects, or unintended and unpredictable, as with uncommon side effects or medical mistakes. Medicine can also cause unintended harm in more subtle ways; it can cause people to worry unnecessarily, for example. 'Healthism', to which I will return later in this chapter, is an unintended outcome of modern medical practice. It can be found in the doctor's consulting room and in the wider world of public health practice. It has the potential to cause harm by making people feel excessively anxious or guilty or be risk-averse or rigid in their behaviour.

It may be more surprising to consider the fact that medical ethics can cause harm, too. The main task of medical ethics is, and has always been, to protect patients and their interests. During recent years it has turned out, however, that medical ethics as a discipline and practice can sometimes be harmful in itself. One way of doing harm is by making patients decide when they would prefer not to decide. Another harm may be caused by the overregulation of research.

In this volume we are taking a long term view of medical care and this chapter focuses on unintended harm as an outcome of medicine as a system and of medical ethics as a discipline and organised practice.

MEDICALISATION REVISITED

> Once upon a time, plenty of children were unruly, some adults were shy, and bald men wore hats. Now all of these descriptions might be attributed to diseases – entities with names, diagnostic criteria, and an increasing array of therapeutic options.[4]

'Medicalisation' has several meanings but it usually refers to the process through which a non-medical problem is defined as a disease or a disorder, or the extension of medical categories in aspects of human lives that were not medical until that moment.[5]

Medicalisation studies became popular in the early 1970s when sociologists began to explore the expanding realm of medicine.[6] Hyperactivity, menopause, post-traumatic stress disorder (PTSD) and alcoholism were among the first medical diagnoses that were analysed critically within this frame of reference.[7] One of the predecessors, Austrian-Mexican theologian and social critic Ivan Illich, had already written about *medical imperialism*, but others saw more complex social forces and processes that could be bi-directional and partial rather than complete.[8] ,

The main focus of medicalisation research in the early years was on the power and authority of the medical profession. The home base for this research has been in sociology but typically medicalisation research goes beyond the borders of sociology of health and stands at the crossroads of ethics, psychology, economics and mass-media studies.[9]

Medicalisation has partly resulted from the secularisation of society. In a way, medicalisation is 'modern theology, a coherent account of beginnings, fallen man, virtue, and divine interventions to those of faith'.[10]

Ivan Illich and medical imperialism

Most radical of the modern critics of medicine was Ivan Illich, who turned his ungracious gaze to medicine, after having written other critical analyses of education and urbanisation. He saw analogical threats in these different areas of life:

> The threat which current medicine represents to the health of populations is analogous to the threat which the volume and intensity of traffic represent to mobility, the threat which education and the media represent to learning, and the threat which urbanisation represents to competence in homemaking.[11]

Illich opened his book on medicine with the now famous claim that the medical establishment had become a major threat to health. He also called for an 'unprecedented housecleaning campaign' among the health professions[12] and an outside assessment of the net contribution of medicine to society's burden of disease.[13]

Illich's analysis was witty:

> Medicine has the authority to label one man's complaint a legitimate illness, to declare a second man sick though he himself does not complain, and to refuse a third social recognition of his pain, his disability, and even his death. It is medicine which stamps some pain as 'merely subjective', some impairment as malingering, and some deaths – though not others – as suicide. ... The judge determines what is legal and who is guilty. The priest declares what is holy and who has broken a taboo. The physician decides what is a symptom and who is sick. He is a moral entrepreneur, charged with inquisitorial powers to discover certain wrongs to be righted.[14]

However, Illich was selective in his documentation and exaggerated shamelessly:

> Organized medicine has practically ceased to be the art of healing the curable, and consoling the hopeless has turned into a grotesque priesthood concerned with salvation and has become a law unto itself.[15]

He was also a romantic and hopelessly partial in some of his analyses. One of the chapter titles in the book speaks for itself: 'Public Controls over the Professional Mafia'.[16] Illich admired traditional cultures that 'made everyone responsible for his own performance under the impact of bodily harm or grief'. In them, 'pain was recognized as an inevitable part of the subjective reality of one's own body in which everyone constantly finds himself, and which is constantly being shaped by his conscious reactions to it'.[17] Illich argued that the technological civilisation starts from opposite assumptions, but his analysis here was thin and references scarce.[18] Sometimes he was just simply wrong:

> The effect of the nocebo, like that of the placebo, is largely independent of what the physician does.[19]

One of Illich's main contributions was his analysis of the different forms that *iatrogenesis* can take. *Iatrogenesis* (from the Greek, meaning 'originating from a physician'):

is clinical when pain, sickness, and death result from medical care; it is social when health policies reinforce an industrial organization that generates ill-health; it is cultural and symbolic when medically sponsored behavior and delusions restrict the vital autonomy of people by undermining their competence in growing up, caring for each other, and aging, or when medical intervention cripples personal responses to pain, disability, impairment, anguish, and death.[20]

Illich wrote his critique on medicine in the early 1970s and he did not live long enough to see that many of his ideas and suggestions are mainstream medical thinking today. Fruitful critical thinking is alive and well *within* medicine today.[21]

Petr Skrabanek and healthism

Case 1. *An elderly woman was worried about her slightly elevated blood pressure. Her GP hesitated but did eventually prescribe medication. A few weeks later the woman fell when she rose up from the ground after a light exercise and fractured her pelvic bone. The causal connection is, of course, uncertain but the point here is the patient was convinced that she needed medication, not the GP.*

Why was this lady so concerned about her blood pressure? When, how and why was she informed that her slightly elevated blood pressure could risk her health? Could she be a victim of the medicalisation of risk factors, in this case a potential risk factor for stroke?

Twenty years after Illich, another witty critic, this time coming from within medicine, began to post short, sharp commentaries on the state of modern medicine to *The Lancet*. Petr Skrabanek was originally from Czechoslovakia but made his career in Dublin, where he and his wife decided to stay when their home country was occupied by the Warsaw Pact troops in 1968.

Skrabanek gave direct credit to Illich for seeing the 'danger of healthism in Western democracies'.[22] The medical monopoly

> deprived people of their autonomy; by supervising and minding them from birth to death (or even from before birth), the art of living and the art of dying, transmitted from generation to generation, were obliterated and lost. The cohesion of traditional communities was replaced by the loneliness of individuals, forming an anonymous mass of 'health consumers'.[23]

Like Illich, Skrabanek seemed to have a romantic view of traditional societies. Unlike Illich, however, he advocated the need for criticism *in* medicine:

> Doctors, aided by scientists, can, by honest admission of ignorance, by demystifying rituals, and by rational inquiry, discover new ways and improve old ways of easing our journey from the cradle to the grave.[24]

Skrabanek supported Western medicine and its rational core but fought against 'a perversion of its ideals, especially in countries dominated by the Anglo-American medical ideology'.[25] He named this enemy *healthism*, an ideology that appeared in Western democracies in the 1970s, having predecessors in the totalitarian ideologies in Nazi Germany and Communist Russia.[26]

He saw a crucial ethical asymmetry between a situation in which a patient knocks at the door of the physician's surgery and shouts, 'Help!', and a situation in which a person in the street is invited for the latest test that is thought to prevent some terrible disease.[27]

Skrabanek found illustrative examples from the mass media, like an interview with a well-known authority on risk factors for heart disease:

> I'm conscious all the time of what fat does to blood cholesterol and that it is fat that mainly puts on fat – so I deliberately avoid chocolate, *which I love* and things such as pies, biscuits, and cakes, which are just stuffed with hidden fat. The one thing, though, that I really miss is sausages. I still *dream* about sausages.[28]

Health terminology is so deeply rooted in our everyday language that even the critics cannot avoid it. According to Skrabanek, 'present-day preoccupations with health are largely unhealthy as the media constantly draw to our attention hazards to health'.[29] He pointed out that most of these hazards are rare, our individual risk of being harmed extremely small, and in this circumstance they should be ignored.

Like Illich, Skrabanek was sometimes selective and disregarded examples that did not support his theses. He cited a German scholar, according to whom, 'prevention based on risk-factor epidemiology is governed by the kind of logic by which room temperature may be lowered by placing the room thermometer into a bucket of ice'.[30] This may sound funny but is clearly false: encouraging infants to sleep on their back to prevent cot death is a simple example of efficient prevention based on risk factor epidemiology only.

For Skrabanek, the risk was that the dominant profession becomes at one and the same time judge, jury and executioner.[31] He argued for a health education that would provide useful, factual information to enhance rational decision making. A potential outcome of such a decision is to ignore the health warning and to accept the risk.

Medicalisation today

The topic of this chapter is unintended harm but, to paint a balanced picture of medicalisation, a few words should be said about its positive aspects. Cataracts, hearing impairment and osteoarthritis are common in old age and perhaps their treatment could be seen as examples of medicalisation, but they significantly improve the quality of life of many people.[32] The medicalisation of death has also brought about palliative medicine and significantly better control of pain and other physical suffering at the end of life.[33]

However, the search for conditions that can be medicalised continues regardless of their significance. 'Overactive bladder syndrome' (OAB) describes a condition that oversimplifies multi-factorial symptoms and implies that OAB is an independent clinical entity with uniform treatment options. According to a recent analysis,[34] the use of the current OAB concept may suppress research endeavouring to understand the underlying causes of OAB symptoms. Another example is attention deficit hyperactivity disorder (ADHD). A recent analysis has demonstrated that American children who are the youngest in their grades are 60% more likely to be diagnosed with ADHD than the oldest children.[35] This analysis suggests that many diagnoses may be driven by teachers' perceptions of poor behaviour among the youngest children in a classroom.

One of the pioneers in the sociology of medicalisation, Peter Conrad, has written about *the shifting engines of medicalisation,* by which he means new forces that drive the process today.[36]

First of these emergent engines has been biotechnology. Pharmaceutical and other biotechnological industries have become major players that have been involved in an increasing amount of public and media promotion. 'Marketing' diseases and promoting genetic tests of potential diseases are just two examples of this. Ideological changes in psychiatry have paved the way for the medicalisation of psychological phenomena.

The role of consumers in the medicalisation process has also grown, and Conrad sees them as another emergent engine. The growth of cosmetic surgery and the activism around adult ADHD, are examples of the expanding role of consumers. The Internet is another phenomenon that may be shifting power from doctors back to people.[37]

Managed care has, according to Conrad, been both a third engine and a constraint in the medicalisation process. It has, for example, reduced insurance coverage for psychotherapy, while being at the same time much more liberal with paying for anti-depressants for example, based on short-term cost considerations.

The discussion and research about medicalisation began with topics related to psychiatry and they are still important today. Critics have argued that the changes in the diagnostic criteria for depression that occurred with the introduction of the Diagnostic and Statistical Manual of the American Psychiatric Association (DSM-III) in 1980 resulted in the treatment of normal emotions of sadness, as well as of depressive disorders. They argued further that contemporary psychiatry has largely ignored the distinction between sadness 'with a cause' and depression 'without cause'.[38] This discussion has become even more vigorous today with the release of DSM-V.[39]

The medicalisation of sexuality is another topic that is as contested today as it was 60 years ago, when the first DSM described 'treatable' behaviours that previously had been seen as morally reprehensible. Homosexuality was now considered a treatable disease, but in 1973 homosexuality was removed from the DSM classification. The success of Viagra, the search for a 'female Viagra' and the use of plastic surgery to produce 'designer vaginas' are examples of the medicalisation of sexuality today.[40]

The association between sexuality and quality of life has been taken seriously by the public health officials, too – sometimes perhaps too seriously. In the early 1990s, Finnish health experts called for 'government-organised sex holidays as a cure for citizens worn down by the stress of modern life'. Petr Skrabanek remarked:

> It might not have occurred to these 'experts' that some of the people they wanted to cure with sexual holidays had been under too much stress from the Finnish health-promotion propaganda against smoking, drinking and sex as causes of cancer.[41]

In addition to medicalisation, *demedicalisation* and even *remedicalisation* of phenomena have also taken place. The demedicalisation of homosexuality has already been mentioned. Circumcision for boys or men is another example of this process: it was demedicalised in the United States, when some social groups reverted to an understanding of circumcision as a religious rather than a health practice.[42] Recently, remedicalisation has taken place because trials have shown that circumcised men are less prone to catching human immunodeficiency virus (HIV) compared with uncircumcised men.

To receive any label, be it only a label as a risk factor, is not insignificant. It has been shown, for example, that the label 'hypertensive' was associated with increased absenteeism because of 'illness' and decreased psychological well-being.[43]

Moynihan *et al.* summarised the harms of medicalisation as follows:

> Inappropriate medicalisation carries the dangers of unnecessary labelling, poor treatment decisions, iatrogenic illness, and economic waste, as well as the opportunity costs that result when resources are diverted away from treating or preventing more serious disease. At a deeper level it may help to feed unhealthy obsessions with health, obscure or mystify sociological or political explanations for health problems, and focus undue attention on pharmacological, individualised, or privatised solutions.[44]

INSTRUMENTAL REASON

Canadian philosopher Charles Taylor describes and analyses three 'malaises of modernity' (or 'sources of worry' in Taylor's own plain English) in his book

The Ethics Of Authenticity.[45] By these he refers to 'features of our contemporary culture and society that people experience as a loss or decline, even as our civilization develops'.

One of the malaises is the primacy of *instrumental reason*, which, for Taylor, means 'the kind of rationality we draw on when we calculate the most economical application of means to a given end'. The worry is that instrumental reason threatens to take over our lives and 'things that ought to be determined by other criteria will be decided in terms of efficiency or "cost–benefit" analysis'. Arguments and considerations that can claim to be based on mathematical thinking or other types of formal calculation have 'great persuasive power in our society, even when this kind of reasoning is not really suited to the subject matter'.

What does this all have to do with medicine and the potential harm caused by it? Consider the following cases:

Case 2. A cost–benefit analysis of amniocentesis to detect chromosomal abnormalities was performed in Denmark. With some preconditions, it was concluded that there was a net benefit to society in providing all pregnant women with amniocentesis.[46]

Case 3. According to a Norwegian study, implementation of the 2003 European guidelines for the prevention of cardiovascular disease in clinical practice would classify most adult Norwegians as having a high risk for fatal cardiovascular disease. For example, at age 50, 40% of the women and 89% of the men were in the high-risk group.[47]

These examples readily demonstrate the power of instrumental reason in contemporary medicine. *Calculative thinking* seems to have spread everywhere in medicine, often at the cost of some important values. Case 2 demonstrates the tension between the two goals of prenatal screening. On the one hand, the goal is to enhance the reproductive autonomy of pregnant women; on the other, the goal is to decrease the number of children born with Down syndrome and save money. It is worth noting that it is no longer politically correct to justify prenatal screening by referring to the latter goal. However, silence about the public health aspect of prenatal screening has not abolished the cost–benefit issue: it is highly improbable that societies would offer prenatal screening without considering the costs.

If Petr Skrabanek were alive, he would undoubtedly make some sarcastic comments about Case 3, where guidelines class most adults in one of the world's longest living and healthiest populations as being at high risk and therefore in need of maximal clinical attention. The authors of the paper conclude that it may be time to reconsider the aims and means of preventing cardiovascular disease and the process of developing guidelines. They also point out that evidence from biomedical research has limited meaning in isolation. Instead, it should be regarded in light of the overall vision, values, strategies and resources that exist in the area of preventive medicine.[48]

Instrumental reason and calculative thinking seem to ignore that every medical decision – be it at the individual or societal level – is made of factual *and* value judgements, and numbers are blind with respect to the latter. Numbers – evidence from scientific studies – are a necessary component of clinical decision making, but even they are not as value-free as one may expect. Molewijk *et al.*[49] demonstrate this in an illustrative study about the development of a decision model for surgery. They conclude that the 'facts have travelled a long, hidden and sometimes arbitrary journey before they are presented as "the facts"'.

That values have importance in decision making is usually acknowledged or taken for granted, but the problems related to their role go unacknowledged. Expressions like 'a patient interprets data regarding risk and can integrate that data into their own system of values'[50] or ' … so they can make informed decisions based on their values'[51] are used as if it would be common to have coherent value systems, into which facts can be integrated. This situation is, however, far from obvious. As Schneider remarks somewhat sarcastically, '[P]eople have better things to do than formulate principles for problems they hope will never arise.'[52]

MEDICAL ETHICS DOING HARM

The main task of medical ethics is to protect patients. By analogy with medicine, it can produce harms, too, but these harms have gone mostly unnoticed. One is a consequence of emphasising the role of autonomy as the leading principle and the other is a result of the ethicalisation of research.

Individualism versus autonomy

One form of malaise that Charles Taylor analyses is *individualism*, which, while being one of the finest achievements of modern civilisation, contains the dark side of 'centring on the self, and a concomitant shutting out, or even unawareness, of the greater issues or concerns that transcend the self, be they religious, political, historical'.[53] This development 'flattens and narrows our lives, makes them poorer in meaning and less concerned with others in society'. 'Modern freedom was won by our breaking loose from older moral horizons. People used to see themselves as part of a larger order.'*

Case 4. *An elderly lady breaks her ankle. At the hospital she has a lengthy discussion with the doctor about the treatment alternatives. The doctor is kind but refuses to decide for the patient. He agrees to decide only after the patient asks him to pretend that she is his mother. The lady happened to be Baroness Mary Warnock, who described the incident a few years later in* The Lancet.[54]

---

* Taylor C. The Ethics Of Authenticity. Cambridge, MA/London: Harvard University Press; 1991. pp. 4, 3.

Case 5. A diagnosis of breast cancer (ductal carcinoma-in-situ) is confirmed for a middle-aged woman. She is given a leaflet containing information about breast cancer and a clinical trial in which she would be randomised to have one of four widely differing treatment options. Within two weeks she should decide about her possible participation in the trial.[55]

Superficially, these examples demonstrate poor communication skills, both in the context of clinical practice and clinical research. However, they also vividly demonstrate the malaise that Taylor describes: individualism. Respect for autonomy has overridden other important values, leading to situations in which patients feel that they have been abandoned. Furthermore, while the formal requirements for informed consent were probably met in Case 5, the actual situation was dealt with in a way that is far from optimal. In the patient's own words: 'The outcome of such a request is to leave the patient feeling isolated at a time when she is much in need of support.'[56]

The expansion of autonomy has made the doctor–patient relationship 'more open, more adult, more transparent, and more attentive to the patient's values and wishes'.[57] At the same time, it has been forgotten that a 'radically independent, autonomous person is at best an idealised portrait of a fictional character, part of an elaborate ideological cartoon of Western culture'.[58] People are, after all, essentially *dependent* beings.[59]

In addition, becoming a patient radically alters the character of personal identity when compared with the normal setting.[60] The so-called 'independent choice' model of decision making, in which physicians objectively present patients with options and odds, but withhold their own experience and recommendations, confuses the concepts of independence and autonomy and assumes that the physician's exercise of power and influence inevitably diminishes the patient's ability to choose freely. It risks sacrificing competence for control, and it discourages active persuasion when differences of opinion exist between the physician and the patient.[61] The obsession with informed consent entails that much of the responsibility falls upon the frail shoulders of the patient.[62] In the name of autonomy, patients may be coerced to make decisions that they may not have made if they had had access to the physician's own opinion about what choices may be best. Loewy has accused autonomy of becoming hidden paternalism that 'abandons patients to their autonomy and makes a relationship which should be mutual and caring, into a cold business transaction'.[63]

Empirical evidence shows that many patients do not wish to make their own medical decisions.[64] Ende *et al.*[65] found that patients prefer that decisions be made principally by their physicians, not themselves, although they very much want to be informed. For most of their patients, the desire to make decisions declined as they faced more severe illness. Older patients had less desire than younger patients to make decisions and to be informed

According to Alfred Tauber, '[M]edical ethics generally, and patient autonomy in particular, filled an ethical lacuna left by the erosion of patient trust, and thus patient autonomy became the sacrosanct principle governing medical ethics'.[66] Onora O'Neill argues: '[C]onceptions of individual autonomy cannot provide a sufficient and convincing starting point for bioethics, or even for medical ethics. They may encourage ethically questionable forms of individualism and self-expression and may heighten rather than reduce public mistrust in medicine, science and biotechnology'.[67] While the minimalist interpretation of individual or personal autonomy in medical ethics fits rather well with medical practice, 'robust conceptions of autonomy may seem a burden and even unachievable for patients; mere choosing may be hard enough'.[68] Erich Loewy, in his paper 'In Defense of Paternalism',[69] maintains that 'the pendulum has swung from rather crass paternalism practised fifty or sixty years ago to an obsession with autonomy which allows patients with questionable autonomy to come to harm'. Eva Feder Kittay[70] goes as far as asking the questions: 'Do we really need the terms paternalism and autonomy? Do they obscure more than they illuminate?'

Ethicalisation of research

Organised ethical review of medical research was launched in the 1970s, following the acceptance of the World Medical Association's Declaration of Helsinki in 1964. There is no doubt that this activity has protected commonly accepted values. There is no evidence, however, that the current regulation process has saved lives or prevented serious harm.

No one is probably against this ethical regulation as such. Recently, however, attention has been paid to possible harm caused by it. A whole conference in 2010 in Uppsala, Sweden, was titled 'Is Medical Ethics Really in the Best Interest of the Patient?'

Ethics regulation has a cost that has received very little attention 'because it slows, discourages and stops life-saving research, lives are lost that would otherwise have been saved'.[71] Only a few attempts have been made to estimate the number of lives lost due to this regulation.

The best and most famous example of an attempt to estimate this was related to the ISIS-2 trial, an international trial of the effect of thrombolytics on the mortality of hospitalised heart attack patients. In the United Kingdom, consent could be obtained by merely mentioning that the patient would be participating in (unspecified) research. In the United States, participants were presented a 1750-word form describing all aspects of the study.[72] This caused delay in the publication of the results and caused, worldwide, 'at least a few thousand unnecessary deaths'.[73]

Ethics regulation may have costs other than those created by delays. Whitney and Schneider summarise these:

That regulation, for example, has sometimes prevented research altogether, which is true of important categories of research in emergency medicine in the United States. Ethics regulation also can affect the quality of research, as when it distorts the representativeness of samples. Ethics regulation may also have a chilling effect that causes researchers not even to attempt some kinds of research. Finally, because many researchers are members of review boards, ethics regulation reduces the time they have to do their own research.[74]

CONCLUDING REMARKS

Medicine and medical ethics needs criticism from both inside and outside. Many times the harm produced by them is not manifest and some effort is needed to make it visible. Although it is difficult and perhaps impossible to quantify some forms of harm, there can be little doubt that the overall balance is positive: both medicine and medical ethics do more good than harm to humankind.

REFERENCES

1. Illich I. *Limits To Medicine. Medical Nemesis: the expropriation of health*. Harmondsworth, Middlesex: Penguin Books; 1976. p. 11.
2. Whitney SN. Estimating the deaths from research regulation. Abstract of a presentation at a conference *Is Medical Ethics Really In the Best Interest of the Patient?*; 2010 14–16 June; Uppsala, Sweden. Available at: www.crb.uu.se/symposia/2010/abstract/whitney.html (accessed 4 August 2013).
3. Loewy E. In defense of paternalism. *Theor Med Bioeth*. 2005; **26**: 445–68.
4. McLellan F. Medicalisation: a medical nemesis. *The Lancet*. 2007; **369**: 627–8.
5. Maturo A. The shifting borders of medicalization: perspectives and dilemmas of human enhancement. In: Maturo A, Conrad P, editors. *The Medicalization Of Life. Salute e Società* No 2; 2009. pp. 13–30.
6. Zola IK. Medicine as an institution of social control. *Sociological Review*. 1972; **20**: 487–504.
7. Conrad P. The shifting engines of medicalization. In: Maturo A, Conrad P, editors. *The Medicalization Of Life. Salute e Società* No 2; 2009. pp. 31–48.
8. Zola IK, op. cit. and Conrad P, op. cit.
9. Maturo A and Conrad P. Introduction. In: Maturo A, Conrad P, editors. *The Medicalization Of Life. Salute e Società* No 2; 2009. pp. 1112.
10. Light DW. Editorial. In: Maturo A, Conrad P, editors. *The Medicalization Of Life. Salute e Società* No 2; 2009. pp. 9–10.
11. Illich I. op. cit. p. 15.
12. Illich I. op. cit. p. 11.
13. Illich I. op. cit. p. 47.
14. Illich I. op. cit. pp. 53–4.
15. Illich I. op cit. p. 249.
16. Illich I. op cit. p. 46.
17. Illich I. op cit. p. 141.

18. Illich I. op cit. p. 142.
19. Illich I. op cit. p. 121.
20. Illich I. op cit. p. 271.
21. For example: Rose S. Beyond medicalisation. *The Lancet.* 2007; **369**: 700–1; Editorial: living with grief. *The Lancet.* 2012; **379**: 589; Macnaughton JM. Medical humanities' challenge to medicine. *Journal of Evaluation in Clinical Practice.* 2011; **17**; 927–32.
22. Skrabanek P. *The Death Of Humane Medicine and the Rise Of Coercive Healthism.* Bury St Edmunds: The Social Affairs Unit; 1994.
23. Skrabanek P. op. cit. p. 17.
24. Skrabanek P, McCormick J. *Follies and Fallacies In Medicine.* New York, NY: Prometheus Books; 1990. p. 9.
25. Skrabanek P. op. cit. p. 12.
26. Skrabanek P. op. cit. p. 11.
27. Skrabanek P. op. cit. p. 36.
28. Skrabanek P. op. cit. p. 69. Emphasis added at first instance; emphasis in original at second instance.
29. Skrabanek P, McCormick J. op cit. p. 44.
30. Skrabanek P. op cit. p. 163.
31. Skrabanek P. op. cit. p. 19.
32. Ebrahim S. The medicalisation of old age should be encouraged. *BMJ.* 2002; **324**: 861–3.
33. Clark D. Between hope and acceptance: the medicalisation of dying. *BMJ.* 2002; **324**: 905–7.
34. Tikkinen KAO, Auvinen A. Does the imprecise definition of overactive bladder serve commercial rather than patient interests? *European Urology.* 2012; **61**: 746–8.
35. Elder TE. The importance of relative standards in ADHD diagnoses: evidence based on exact birth dates. *Journal of Health Economics.* 2010; **29**: 641–56.
36. Conrad P.
37. Moynihan R, Smith R. Too much medicine? *BMJ.* 2002; **324**: 859–60.
38. Horwitz AV, Wakefield JC. The medicalization of sadness: how psychiatry transformed a natural emotion into a mental disorder. In Maturo A, Conrad P, editors. *The Medicalization Of Life. Salute e Società* No 2; 2009. pp. 49–66.
39. Light DW. op. cit.
40. Hart G, Wellings K. Sexual behaviour and its medicalisation: in sickness and in health. *BMJ.* 2002; **324**: 896–900.
41. Skrabanek P. op. cit. p. 108.
42. Carpenter LM. Demedicalization and remedicalization of male circumcision in Great Britain and the United States. In: Maturo A, Conrad P, editors. *The Medicalization Of Life. Salute e Società* No 2. 2009; pp. 155–71.
43. Haynes RB, Sackett DL, Taylor DW, *et al.* Increased absenteeism from work after detection and labeling of hypertensive patients. *N Engl J Med.* 1978; **299**: 741–4.
44. Moynihan R, Heath I, Henry D. Selling sickness: the pharmaceutical industry and disease mongering. *BMJ.* 2002; **324**: 886–91.
45. Taylor C. *The Ethics Of Authenticity.* Cambridge, MA/London: Harvard University Press; 1991. pp. 1, 5.
46. Goldstein H, Philip J. A cost–benefit analysis of prenatal diagnosis by amniocentesis in Denmark. *Clin Genet.* 1990; **37**: 241–63.

47. Getz L, Sigurdsson JA, Hetlevik I, *et al.* Estimating the high risk group for cardiovascular disease in the Norwegian HUNT 2 population according to the 2003 European guidelines: modelling study. *BMJ.* 2005; **331**: 551–5.
48. Getz, *et al.* op. cit.
49. Molewijk AC, Stiggelbout AM, Otten W, *et al.* Implicit normativity in evidence-based medicine: a plea for integrated empirical ethics research. *Health Care Anal.* 2003; **11**: 69–92.
50. Editorial. Making the 'right' health care decisions: why values matter. *PLoS Med.* 2009; **6**(8 August): e1000136. doi: 10.1371/journal.pmed.1000136.
51. Punales Morejon D. Society's diseases [commentary]. *Hastings Cent Rep.* 1996; **26**: 21–2.
52. Schneider CE. Some realism about informed consent. *J Lab Clin Med.* 2005; **145**: 289–91.
53. Taylor C. op. cit. p. 14.
54. Warnock M. An attack on the autonomy of patients (book review). *The Lancet.* 2009; **374**: 1137–8.
55. Thornton HM. Breast cancer trials: a patient's viewpoint. *The Lancet.* 1992; **339**: 44–5.
56. Thornton HM. op. cit.
57. Pellegrino E. Physician integrity: why it is inviolable. In: Crowley, M., editor. *Connecting American Values with Health Reform.* Garrison, NY: Hastings Center; 2009. pp. 18–20. Available at: www.thehastingscenter.org/Publications/Detail.aspx?id=3528
58. Tauber AI. *Patient Autonomy and the Ethics of Responsibility.* Cambridge, MA/London: MIT Press; 2005.
59. Nys T, Denier Y, Vandevelde T. Introduction. In: Nys T, Denier Y, Vandevelde T, editors. *Autonomy & Paternalism. Reflections On the Theory and Practice Of Health Care.* Leeuven: Peeters; 2007. pp. 1–22.
60. Tauber AI. op. cit.
61. Quill TE, Brody H. Physician recommendations and patient autonomy: finding a balance between physician power and patient choice. *Ann Intern Med.* 1996; **125**: 763–9.
62. Nys, *et al.* op. cit.
63. Loewy E. op. cit.
64. Schneider CE.
65. Ende J, Kazis L, Ash A, *et al.* Measuring patients' desire for autonomy: decision-making and information-seeking preferences among medical patients. *J Gen Intern Med.* 1989; 4: 23–30.
66. Tauber AI. op. cit. p. 5.
67. O'Neill O. *Autonomy and Trust In Bioethics.* Cambridge: Cambridge University Press; 2002. p. 73.
68. O'Neill O. op. cit. p. 38.
69. Loewy E. op. cit.
70. Kittay EF. Beyond autonomy and paternalism. In: Nys T, Denier Y, Vandevelde T, editors. *Autonomy & Paternalism: reflections on the theory and practice of health care.* Leeuven: Peeters; 2007. pp. 23–70.
71. Whitney SN, Schneider CE. A method to estimate the cost in lives of ethics board review of biomedical research. *Journal of Internal Medicine.* 2011; **269**: 392–406.
72. Whitney SN, Schneider CE. op. cit.
73. Whitney SN and Schneider CE. op. cit.
74. Whitney SN and Schneider CE. op. cit.

9

Technology, ageing and death

IONA HEATH

PROGNOSIS: AGEING, TECHNOLOGY AND DEATH

Young and old

The editor and writer Diana Athill has become the great contemporary chronicler of the regrets, compensations and pleasures of old age. In her 2002 book *Yesterday Morning*, published when she was 85, she writes:

> The big event of old age – the thing which replaces love and creativity as a source of drama – is death.[1]

The older a person gets, the less he or she needs a doctor to define the prognosis. Unlike most young people, most older people are quite accepting of the finitude of their lives and they have an increasingly clear experiential understanding of the multiple processes by which the body, cumulatively, lets them down, becoming an ever-increasing liability so that eventually they will be content to shuffle it off. Dylan Thomas acknowledged that 'wise men at their end know dark is right'[2] while perversely urging his father to 'rage, rage against the dying of the light'. He illustrates how different the perspective of relatives, like Geoff's daughter Mary in our stories, can be from that of an old person like Geoff who knows he is dying or has nothing more to live for. Too often, relatives and perhaps especially grown children, attempt to show their love by insisting that the dying and their doctors struggle on.

In his poem about a hospital entitled 'The Building', Philip Larkin writes:

> All know they are going to die.
> Not yet, perhaps not here, but in the end,
> And somewhere like this.[3]

However, most doctors are not old and most lack the existential wisdom of the old. Indeed young doctors are often lucky enough to be still in life's immortal phase and perhaps cannot be expected to understand what it is to know that death is sure to come within the next few years or even months or weeks. However, this lack of understanding has consequences. The Dutch physician Bert Keizer, writing about the death of his own father in 2001, noted that:

> One of the most ill-starred meetings in modern medicine is that between a frail, defenceless old man nearing the end of his life, and an agile young intern at the beginning of his career.[4]

Young doctors are also influenced by current social expectations. The medical historian Charles Rosenberg asks:

> How does one manage death – which is not precisely a disease – when demands for technological ingenuity and activism are almost synonymous with public expectations of a scientific medicine?[5]

For me, this is one of the most serious challenges facing doctors in the richer countries of the world who find themselves caring for an increasingly elderly population. The Office for National Statistics (ONS) predicts that a third of the babies born in 2012 will live for more than 100 years.[6]

Technological activism

Excessive technological activism has a long history. In a letter to his mother written in 1890, Anton Chekhov, physician and writer, expressed a common discomfort:

> On the road I examined a man with cancer of the liver. The man was emaciated and hardly breathing, but this did not deter the medical assistant from putting twelve cupping glasses on him.[7]

There are many more recent examples of futile medical interventions at the end of life. Samuel Beckett's *Malone Dies* is perhaps the most authentic memento mori of our own time:

> And when they cannot swallow any more someone rams a tube down their gullet, or up their rectum, and fills them full of vitaminized pap, so as not to be accused of murder.[8]

This was written more than 60 years ago, which equates to at least two medical generations, and it is disturbing to consider how much truer it has become over the intervening years. It is all too easy for doctors to retreat from their patients into inappropriate medical activism because

> [p]hysicians are thrust repeatedly into situations in which the *professional* tasks peculiar to their status as physicians are linked to the *existential* tasks they share with all persons: maintaining a sense of meaning, security, and connectedness in the face of mortality and finitude.[9]

The fundamental problem is that physicians have neither any particular aptitude nor any relevant education in facing these shared and intensely difficult existential tasks; they have no grounding in the philosophy that has helped people to grapple with the threat of mortality over millennia and little knowledge of the profoundly dignified and comforting assertions first by Epicurus and then by Lucretius that:

> Death is nothing to us. When we exist death is not, and when death exists we do not.[10]

Sentiments echoed in the Epicurean epitaph:

> *Non fui, fui, no sum, non curo.* (I was not, I was, I am not, I care not.)

Michel de Montaigne owned a copy of Lucretius's verse essay 'On the Nature of Things' and he quotes from it more than 100 times in his own *Essays*.[11] In the margin of his 1563 edition of Lucretius' poem, he wrote:

> Fear of death is the cause of all our vices.

And this seems particularly true of the vices of modern medicine, which allow doctors and other healthcare professionals to pretend that, to a very great extent, death is nothing to do with them. This leads directly either to the imposition of inappropriate and futile treatments at the end of life or to ignoring the predicament and the needs of the dying by failing to acknowledge or even recognise them.

Atul Gawande, the American surgeon and *New Yorker* columnist, writes:

> In the past few decades, medical science has rendered obsolete centuries of experience, tradition, and language about our mortality, and created a new difficulty for mankind: how to die. People die only once. They have no experience to draw upon. They need doctors and nurses who are willing to have the hard

discussions and say what they have seen, who will help people prepare for what is to come – and to escape a warehoused oblivion that few really want.[12]

But it is intensely difficult to have hard discussions and the most needed ones are perhaps the hardest of all.

Selling sickness

Hegel anticipated our contemporary situation with telling insight:

> What the English call 'comfort' is something inexhaustible and illimitable. Others can reveal to you that what you take to be comfort at any stage is discomfort, and these discoveries never come to an end. Hence the need for greater comfort does not exactly arise within you directly; it is suggested to you by those who hope to make a profit from its creation.[13]

The aspiration to postpone death indefinitely has become a form of comfort suggested and promoted by those who also hope to make a profit from its creation. More recently, Ivan Illich has developed Hegel's argument and his predictions are proving uncomfortably accurate.

> The more time, toil and sacrifice spent by a population in producing medicine as a commodity, the larger will be the by product, namely the fallacy that society has a supply of health locked away which can be mined and marketed.[14]

The market imperative is that only a minority of most populations is acutely ill at any one time whereas the majority of most populations are healthy. The healthy are, however, susceptible to persuasion that it is necessary for them to optimise their prognosis by undergoing screening and/or by taking preventive medication. Those older people who are relatively well seem to be no less susceptible to this persuasion. And, in affluent countries, because there is now more money to be made from selling so-called 'healthcare' interventions for the healthy majority than for the sick minority, there is more pharmaceutical research in pursuit of preventive treatments than for the treatment of those who are already sick.[15]

As a direct result, society spends an ever greater amount on preventive technologies, leaving less available to treat those who are actually sick. In so doing, we shift resources from the poor and the sick to the rich and the well. This is clearly good for the medical technology and pharmaceutical industries but very bad for those funding the healthcare system, particularly as preventive technologies are much more likely to prove futile and to be overtaken by other disasters or pathologies.

The 2002 PROSPER study provides a cogent example.[16] It is one of the very few studies of cardiovascular prevention in older people and is a trial of the effects of pravastatin in elderly individuals assessed to be at risk of cardiovascular disease. More than 5000 participants, aged 70 to 82 years, were followed up for an average of 3.2 years. The results of the trial showed that pravastatin did indeed reduce rates of fatal and non-fatal myocardial infarction and stroke. However, all-cause mortality was unchanged and rates of cancer diagnosis and cancer death were higher in the treatment group. There is no suggestion that statins cause cancer but, by closing off one cause of death, others are inevitably opened – first cancer, and then dementia.[17] This exemplifies an unprecedented contemporary phenomenon. When we vaccinate children in infancy, we are selecting out a cause of death for them, in this case justifiably, because deaths from infectious diseases tend to occur prematurely. However, when we select out causes of death for people who have already exceeded the average lifespan, the whole endeavour becomes morally questionable. How often when we as doctors offer a statin to an elderly patient do we seek genuinely informed consent? Most older people would accept such a medication if they were told that it would reduce their chances of dying of a heart attack or a stroke, but if the doctor went on to tell them that the medication would not help them to live any longer and would increase their chances of being diagnosed with cancer or dementia, how many would still want it?

A more recent study underlines the prevalence of futility within healthcare today. Researchers at the Veterans Health Administration in the United States set out to measure the prevalence of statin use during the last six months of life and to determine if statin prescribing varied according to the presence of a recognisable, life-limiting condition.[18] They identified 3031 patients who died during the calendar year 2004 and within that group they found that 1584 (52%) were taking statin medication during the last six months of life. They then identified 337 of these 1584 who had a diagnosed terminal condition and they compared this group with controls who did not have such a diagnosis but were matched for age, socioeconomic status and number of comorbidities. Shockingly, there was no significant difference in the time off statins between the cases and the controls. The authors concluded that their findings demonstrated a missed opportunity to reduce the therapeutic burden on dying patients and to limit healthcare spending.

Therapeutic burden

In Chapter 5 John Saunders draws our attention to the painting entitled *Self Portrait: Between Clock and Bed*, which was painted between 1940 and 1942. Munch was in his late 70s at the time and like Geoff in our stories, is caught between the clock and the bed, between the vertical and the horizontal. In this situation, open, rational discussions and mutually responsible decisions about the point at which medicine becomes futile and wasteful are fundamentally important. There seems to be huge reluctance among doctors and policymakers to discuss any of this, which is all too easy to understand because such discussions are often difficult and painful. Nonetheless, the reluctance is regrettable, especially when accusations of ageism are used to mask increasingly futile interventions that verge on cruelty.

When the prognosis is limited by age and infirmity, time is a precious commodity not to be wasted on the routines and rituals of modern medical care. Carl May and colleagues have proposed the concept of 'minimally disruptive medicine'.[19] They conclude that the 'work' of being sick is made more onerous by serial advances in diagnosis and treatment. They illustrate their argument with several examples, one of which is:

> A man being treated for heart failure in UK primary care rejected the offer to attend a specialist heart failure clinic to optimise management of his condition. He stated that in the previous two years he had made 54 visits to specialist clinics for consultant appointments, diagnostic tests, and treatment. The equivalent of one full day every two weeks was devoted to this work.

Doctors may be blighting many older people's lives by allowing diagnostic categories to dominate, determine and standardise the ways in which we care for illness and attempt to relieve suffering. Charles Rosenberg writes about the 'tyranny of diagnosis':

> Specific disease categories are omnipresent at the beginning of the 21st century, playing substantive roles in a variety of contexts and interactions ranging from the definition and management of deviance to the disciplining of practitioners and the containment of hospital costs.

The rhetoric of care pathways, payment by results, unacceptable variation and much else prevails. Where is the wisdom that medicine so urgently needs?

A fair innings

The eighteenth-century English poet William Cowper was himself a patient with recurrent mental health problems and a history of a serious suicide attempt. In 'The Task', he wrote these lines:

> Knowledge and wisdom, far from being one,
> Have oftimes no connexion. Knowledge dwells
> In heads replete with thoughts of other men;
> Wisdom in minds attentive to their own.
> Knowledge, a rude unprofitable mass,
> The mere material with which Wisdom builds,
> Till smooth'd and square'd, and fitted to its place,

Does not encumber what it means to enrich.
Knowledge is proud that he has learn'd so much,
Wisdom is humble that he knows no more.[20]

The wisdom we seek often resides within our older patients if we would but listen. In 1997, the health economist Alan Williams, then in his 70s and now dead, courageously proposed that healthcare should be rationed by age using what he described as the 'fair innings' argument. His conviction was that:

> This attempt to wring the last drop of medical benefit out of the system, no matter what the human and material costs, is not the hallmark of a humane society. In each of our lives there has to come a time when we accept the inevitability of death, and when we also accept that a reasonable limit has to be set on the demands we can properly make on our fellow citizens in order to keep us going a bit longer.[21]

Williams argued that a good start to defining a fair innings would be the biblical definition of three score years and ten. It is a pleasing coincidence that Diana Athill, writing when she was more than 90 years of age, reports that for her old age began at 71.[22] Scottish poet John Burnside captures the subtlety of the ageing body in lines from his poem 'The Gravity Chair':

> I was seven, or seventeen, and I didn't know
> how ageing works, like Zeno's paradox,
> adjusting all the time, to right itself;
>
> yet sometimes, on a winter afternoon,
> I thought of someone skilled – a juggler, say –
> adapting to the pull of gravity
>
> by shifts and starts, till something in the flesh
> – a weightedness, a plumb-line to the earth –
> revealed itself, consenting to be still.[23]

Alongside its subtlety, there is a potential kindness in ageing that was recognised by Joseph Roth in the dying days of the Austro-Hungarian Empire:

> The infirmities of old age are a blessing. Forgetfulness, deafness and failing eyesight as we grow old, and a little confusion before death. The shadows it casts before it are cool and kindly.[24]

We need this sort of wisdom and yet it is everywhere threatened. If we are prepared to listen to what old people tell us, we hear about the slow attrition of their generation that eventually reaches a tipping point when spouse and almost all friends have died, and even offspring and their generation are beginning to die. The endless sequence of losses shifts the balance of fear and resignation. Through this process, old people seem to become less afraid of the 'when' of death but they remain afraid of the 'how'. At any age it is difficult to die and it is difficult to watch others die: the physical body often seems to have an enormous will to live that may prolong the distress of dying.

Yet as people get older, high-tech interventional and invasive care becomes less acceptable to them. How many elderly patients tell their doctors that they will never again agree to go into hospital? At the same time, intimate, tender, physical care becomes proportionately more important. Yet, as a society, we have devalued intimate physical care and many nurses now seem over-qualified to deliver it. Computers displace care and treatment mediated by touch and listening:

> Few of the tragedies at life's end are as rending to the clinician as that of the frail elderly patient who has no one to tell the life story to. Indeed, becoming a surrogate for those who should be present to listen may be one of the practitioner's finest roles in the care of the aged.[25]

One of the great pleasures of general practice is the opportunity to hear the stories of those patients who were alive long before we were even born – every one of them in some way extraordinary.

Inevitability

The contemporary Dutch philosopher Annemarie Mol seems to follow in a long tradition that is captured in the title of one of Montaigne's essays: To philosophise is to learn how to die.[26] Mol spent time observing the care given to patients attending a hospital diabetic clinic in the Netherlands. She describes processes of care that are sensitive, patient, pragmatic and iterative and that never lose sight of the fact that the final task of medicine is the care of the dying. She writes:

> You do what you can, you try and try again. You doctor, but you have no control. And ultimately the result is not glorious: stories about life with a disease do not end up with everybody 'living happily ever after'. They end with death.[27]

> Diseases are erratic, so good doctors do not make promises. There is only one certainty: in the end, you die. The moment will be different for each of us, but that it will come is certain. … In the logic of care there is a limit to activism.

There seems an urgent need to rediscover traditions of resignation, stoicism and courage in the face of death on the part of both the dying and those who love and care for them. We need better ways of coping with the pain that comes with the loss of life and love. The Canadian novelist Robertson Davies who, like Chekhov and Gawande was both a writer and a doctor, noted:

> As so often, I thought that the real heroism of death was seen in the one who stood by.[28]

We have allowed long traditions of ritual to wither away with the religions that underpinned them but, at the same time, we have lost the framework of behaviour that ritual provided and the comfort and security that this can bring. People feel adrift and uncertain and have little idea of what is expected of them.

The calm of too many deaths is sabotaged by ill-considered attempts at cardiopulmonary resuscitation (CPR) because, whenever an ambulance is called to a collapsed patient, the paramedics are instructed to attempt CPR. Older patients and their relatives have a right to know the likely result. In the optimal circumstances of resuscitation within hospital, only 17% of patients, across the age range, survive to be discharged and of these only 51% are well enough to return home.[29] The older the patient, the smaller the possibility of benefit, and so, as with any other invasive healthcare intervention, should patients not be invited to opt in, rather than being required to opt out? Current practice creates yet another scenario within contemporary medicine where the small chance of benefit for the few creates procedures that risk the peace and dignity of the many.

Finding meaning

Mary Midgeley, another contemporary philosopher, writes:

> [S]ince people's deepest ideas about the meaning or meaninglessness of life are largely forged in everyday life and in the arts, we would surely do well to pay serious attention to these wherever we can find them.[30]

For doctors, our patients are our great resource of everyday life, and we also have the arts. The critic and writer James Wood elucidates the place of literature:

> Literature can no more 'explain' suffering than can science or religion, but it can describe it better than either. If great suffering forces theology into embarrassed silence and atheism into cocksure noise, it prompts literature to measured lament, which is all we have right now.[31]

Pain, suffering, resignation, loss and fear all circulate around the ultimate and universal prognosis at the end of life. Writers and perhaps particularly poets face these issues both more obliquely and more directly. They use words with care, thought and deliberation to approach a truth that is recognised by others with an immediacy that makes them feel less alone. Aspects of our experience of life and the world have been acknowledged and described. The greatest poets reveal truths that we as readers already know but with a new clarity and a new depth that enriches and extends our understanding of our own experience of the 'million petalled flower of being here'.[32]

Diana Athill, finding herself 'somewhere towards the end', suggests that it may yet be possible to delight in the present and leave the prognosis to look after itself.

REFERENCES

1. Athill D. *Yesterday Morning*. London: Granta Books; 2002.
2. Thomas D. Do not go gentle into that good night. In: *Collected Poems 1934–1953*. London: JM Dent; 1998 (1951).
3. Larkin P. The building. In: *Collected Poems*. London: Faber and Faber Limited; 1988 (1972).
4. Keizer B. Living well, dying well. In: *Medicine and Humanity*. London: King's Fund; 2001.
5. Rosenberg CE. The tyranny of diagnosis: specific entities and individual experience. *The Milbank Quarterly*. 2002; **80**(2): 237–60.
6. Office for National Statistics (ONS). *What Are the Chances of Surviving To Age 100?* London: ONS; 2012.
7. Chekhov A. Letter from Siberia, 1890. Quoted in Coope J. *Dr Chekhov: a study in literature and medicine*. Cross Publishing; 1997.
8. Beckett S. *Malone Dies*. London: Penguin Books, 1962 (1951).
9. Barnard D. Love and death: existential dimensions of physicians' difficulties with moral problems. *J Med Philos*. 1988; **13**: 393–409.
10. Long AA, Sedley DN. *The Hellenistic Philosophers*. Cambridge: Cambridge University Press; 1987.
11. Greenblatt S. *The Swerve: how the world became modern*. New York, NY: WW Norton & Company; 2011.
12. Gawande A. Letting go. *New Yorker*. 27 July 2010.
13. Hegel GW. *Elements of the Philosophy of Right*; 1822.
14. Illich I. *Limits to Medicine*. London: Marion Boyars Publishers; 1975.
15. Freemantle N, Hill S. Medicalisation, limits to medicine, or never enough money to go around? *BMJ*. 2002; **324**: 864–5.
16. Shepherd J, Blauw GJ, Murphy MB, *et al*. Pravastatin in elderly individuals at risk of vascular disease (PROSPER): a randomised controlled trial. *The Lancet*. 2002; **360**: 1623–30.
17. Mangin D, Sweeney K, Heath I. Preventive health care in elderly people needs rethinking. *BMJ*. 2007; **335**: 285–7.
18. Silveira MJ, Kazanis AS, Shevrin MP. *J Palliat Med*. 2008; **11**: 685–93.
19. May C, Montori V, Mair F. We need minimally disruptive medicine. *BMJ*. 2009; **339**: b2803, doi: 10.1136/bmj.b2803.

20. Cowper W. *The Task*; 1785.
21. Williams A. The rationing debate: rationing health care by age. *BMJ*. 1997; **314**: doi: 10.1136.
22. Athill D. *Somewhere Towards the End*. London: Granta Books; 2008.
23. Burnside J. *The Gravity Chair*; 2002.
24. Roth J. *The Emperor's Tomb*; 1938.
25. Kleinman A. *Illness Narratives*; 1988.
26. de Montaigne M. To philosophize is to learn how to die. In: *The Complete Essays*; 1: 20.
27. Mol A. *The Logic Of Care: health and the problem of patient choice*; 2006.
28. Davies R. *The Cunning Man*; 1994.
29. www.mcw.edu/FileLibrary/User/jrehm/fastfactpdfs/Concept179.pdf (accessed 23 April 2012).
30. Midgeley M. *Science As Salvation: a modern myth and its meaning*; 1992.
31. Wood J. Sea changes. *The Guardian Review*. Saturday 22 January 2005.
32. Larkin P. *The Old Fools*; 1973.

10

Open futures, human finitude

MARTYN EVANS

Frail as summer's flower we flourish
Blows the wind and it is gone
Yet while mortals rise and perish
God endures unchanging on.
Henry Francis Lyte

In the long run we are all dead.
John Maynard Keynes

INTRODUCTION

'Looking forward' is an ambiguous state in which to find oneself, as ambiguous as that future reality of which the looking-forward is a presentiment. Anticipation can be eager and excited (cats are said to enjoy the prospect of food as much as the food itself), but it can also be fearful (for instance, contemplation supplies the frightened soldier with full-dress-rehearsals of his death). For context is all. Prognosis usually concerns where illness may take us and where it may leave us. Often this can be entirely happy: the full recovery with years of active future life restored or confirmed. Or it can be sombre: striking the tempo of the introductory bars to an elegy for life diminished, darkened or soon-to-be-lost altogether.

Prognosis is a coolly-anticipatory dipping of the toe into time's cold stream, best-guessing what the full plunge will be like. Of course its roots proclaim prognosis as fore-*knowing*. But there is something bordering on the contradictory in that idea: we know backwards; we rarely know forwards. More modestly, as a form of attempted fore-*seeing*, prognosis searches out glimpsed stages in the lived measures of time: becoming, fully being, diminishing, finishing. Its assumptions place disease, illness, recovery or decline within the usual course of uninterrupted life; and that course in turn consists in the single stanza of an imagined chorale, whose individual lines vary with our lives, but whose line-endings are ordinarily the same:

Furnish : Relish : Languish : Perish

Later on, I will return to the musical metaphor; but in introducing it one may be tempted to remark, as does Fingarette, that 'Confucius's vision of human life may be helpful to us because it compensates for a characteristic blindness from which we modern Westerners suffer – our blindness to the ceremonial dimension of social existence'.[1] This is perhaps not entirely fair; in Western Christendom chorales have for centuries expressed the measured tread of worshippers' relationships with one another as well as with the eternal. But while our ceremonial forms, such as they are, inspire us to make selected words in some sense more present to us through music, those words' meanings are typically attenuated rather than vivified in the process. The body – and let us not forget for a moment that prognosis is more securely tied to processes written within the body than it is to our experience of those processes – responds to and exhibits music more readily than words. One is reminded here of Wackenroder's observation, quoted by Spitzer, that:

> Seasons, times of day, lives and destinies, are all, strikingly enough, thoroughly rhythmical, metrical, according to a beat. In all trades and arts, in all machines, in organic bodies, in our daily functions, everywhere: rhythm, meter, beat, melody.[2]

But whether in prose or in music, the scale of our line-endings is normally too large for us to take in; instead we mark out the ground-metre of ordinary living in more manageable and prosaic ways. Often words do this well enough. Recall our patient Jen through the calendar she kept, upon which a chorale might readily be hung:

> Siskins today. Saw the wren! Visited Geoff.
> Hospital today. Dr Friend.
> Woodpecker. First this year.
> *Woodpecker. First this year.*

Whatever their scale, the watermark of mortality runs through these plangent lines, through every event, every heartbeat. But mortality also implies life in every heartbeat. Perhaps it is just as well that it does. For whether by temperament, or because life has to be lived in the present, we are generally only dimly aware of the larger stanzas, or of the life-celebrating chorale as a whole. In this chapter I would like to indulge our being thus 'dimly aware', for a little while.

I – THE OPENNESS OF THE FUTURE

We cannot see the future, although we can peer towards it. This is important for our present reflections because prognosis is, after all, future-orientated. We expect that, in the most general terms concerning the way the material world behaves, the future will resemble the past. Reasonably so; however, this expectation is limited in two ways. First, our understanding of the material world is highly incomplete, and the gaps affect our understanding of disease processes, of the full range of factors at stake in giving rise to them, and of different human bodies' sometimes bafflingly variable responses to them. Second, our understanding of the material world can take only limited account of how our own actions and intentions and purposes affect future events – not least because we ourselves do not know precisely what we will do. My intention this afternoon was to complete a substantial portion of this very chapter during a period of time I had scheduled to devote to the task, and at lunchtime that prospect seemed a real one. It was overturned the moment that an unexpected knock at the door brought an equally unexpected problem with which I had to deal. Of course, this is the stuff of daily life: negotiated action, deferred intentions, unanticipated joyful encounters, the springing up of hidden obstacles or dangers, the fallibility of our bodies, our seemingly infinite distractibility. It has been said that the past is 'another country'. Perhaps the future, so far as we can peer into it, is a land of possibilities of which some will come to pass in ways that we can deliberately influence – but can rarely control.

The future is undetermined by the past, then, and also by the present: it is 'open' in a way that the past is not, nor even the rolling present, in which we continually act only to see those actions become instantly irretrievable – for all that we can often amend or mitigate their consequences. But the future is not *boundlessly* open. There are some things that simply cannot happen, some possibilities that are forever excluded. Jake can recall the moment at which his relationship with his first love, Carol, stood on a cusp – to bond, or to fissure – but he cannot *retrieve* it in order that he may now choose differently. I can never again lead the life of a young enquirer still at the point of discovering philosophical reflection with its entire repertoire of investigations, among which I could choose my speciality; I can never again look into a mirror and see the reflection of that hirsute, awkward youth whose cocky spirit somehow still 'inhabits' me in pale and complicated ways. (Or as Joni

Mitchell famously observed, no one could ever say to Van Gogh, 'Paint *A Starry Night* again, man.'[†]). This at least we can know of the future.

And some things cannot happen *yet*. Processes of maturation – physical and existential alike – cannot be rushed, even when we can see to what they will lead. Patients may surprise us in the rate, as well as the extent, to which they can recover or be rehabilitated, but physical recovery takes time and emotional recovery may be circumscribed. If Rachel's becoming a mother is really ever to stabilise her self-management of her insulin it will be from a future perspective that we can know it, not from the present.

Prognosis has an intriguing relationship with hindsight. It is based (loosely, and with awkward philosophical reservations concerning induction[3]) upon our accumulating experiences, and particularising onto a known individual the general expectations arising from collectedly observed patients in the past. In that sense it rests upon hindsight. At the same time it defies hindsight because it gazes ahead, in either hope or discouragement as the case suggests. We can 'read' the patient's life backwards, guessing at the causes and the reasons, the genes and the choices, that led to the present diagnosis – and to the need for the present prognosis. We cannot similarly 'read' the patient's life forwards, except possibly in the most grievous cases where the clockwork of life's end-stage is already running down (or running awry) beyond the point of meaningful intervention.

Hindsight, moreover, is the reading of a history of possibilities foreclosed. 'With hindsight we might have acted differently,' we commonly say – but it is never true in any meaningful sense, because *at the time* what we needed was not hindsight at all, but foresight. The fact is that we begin life with possibilities that, for the most part, diverged precisely because they excluded one another. One cannot be both the child who took up piano lessons and the child who did not. There was a point in time from which even to take up lessons a single week later is to become a different child: the child whose previous week has an irretrievably different history – and a different future influence – from the child who began at once. The differences may be indiscernible yet they accumulate. Our possibilities are added to as life proceeds: opportunities come our way and we take them or decline them as the case may be. We enact a growing, and bewildering, variety of new potentials – physical and social and intellectual and emotional.

And yet every choice and every 'enacting' excludes some other choices and acts; the 'road not taken' is testament to the road we actually chose. Our lives' futures begin as, seemingly, illimitably broad potential and at a distance that from the child's perspective appears unattainably distant. Yet a long heartbeat later and we are already looking back on a life largely accomplished. There are

---

† In a recorded aside between songs, on her live album *Miles of Aisles*, Warner Music: Elektra/ Asylum Records, 1974.

many tracks we may trace across our futures, but there can be only one track that, in the event, we did trace. Walking past what she takes to be the accusatory gaze of others, Rachel's conviction that 'she'd never escape the curiosity in those eyes' is itself a kind of existential prognosis arising from her dawning sense of responsibility, one tied to her actions in the moment quite as securely as her medical prognosis is tied to her diabetes. And from that moment forward she carries both with her. Our present moments are the convergences of all that we in fact did – but also the divergences of all that we yet may do. The present is a lens, magnifying a moving point across a map: in front of it, a conjectural plot; behind it, an ineradicable trace. The future both opens out to us and closes upon us; over time, the closing down, the subtraction, can seem to dominate us. As we grow older, and as less time remains to us, then the convergences increasingly outweigh the divergences. Habit's hand grasps us more tightly; shaking free (perhaps even wanting to shake free) becomes steadily less possible.

But perhaps this is true more in a quantitative sense (the number, extent and duration of distinct opportunities) than in a qualitative sense. The moments remaining to us may become individually richer, more nuanced and more meaningful as they dwindle in sheer number. The musical phrasing of our lives begins in crescendo, and at some later time ends in diminuendo; yet life, like music, can intensify in the quietening simplicity of a coda's concluding bars, and there are some very long and rich codas in music and life alike.

II – DEFYING OUR FINITUDE

The constraints upon the openness of the future are doubly poignant. Every choice taken is a multitude of other choices forgone, but in an illimitable ocean of lifespan this might not matter: the chief decision facing us would concern the order in which to undertake things, rather than which things we had time to undertake. But that possibility is denied us by our own finitude – the unpredictable yet unopposable limitations upon both our powers and the time available to us in which to exercise them. Acknowledging our finitude is the first step on the path of coming to terms with it, and prognosis in illness is an effective prompt to do so.

Now the acknowledgement of finitude may confront many facets. Most obviously, there is the finitude of our just *being* – of our essential mortality (which prognosis always implicitly attempts to meter). Because mortality is essential to us, it is part of the meaning of 'being human'. Thus it is more than simply our vulnerability: some humans are more vulnerable than others, but none is more or less mortal than anyone else. This finitude in turn points to others. Our material being is certainly delimited, but it is imperfectly defined; the space our bodies occupy is co-inhabited, by ourselves and by the countless microorganisms that live on and in us.[4] We metamorphose continuously –

gently over a day or a week, brutally over a lifetime. Even within its general envelope, our spatial finitude is malleable in detail – malleable by ourselves (as when by effort and will we purposefully develop our muscles) and malleable by disease processes of atrophy or neoplasia (as when cancer replaces cells that are 'us' with cells that are 'not-us').

Of course, it is a difficult thing simply to *be*: generally we *are* through how we engage with the world, be it actively or in contemplation. So (particularly in Western culture where our instincts for action ahead of contemplation form something of a fetish) it is salutary to remember the finitude of our *acting* – our portions of strength, stamina, talent and fortitude which will all one day run out and which must somehow be expended adventurously while also husbanded against the foreseeable needs of our later decline, what Larkin calls 'the coming night'.[5] The fatally unadventurous Jake has plenty of time for contemplation and action alike. He is a prisoner, not only (as he imagines) of his psoriasis, but (in truth) of his habits – 'His hands were good now, but old habits died hard' – in which habits of self-loathing and self-deprecation, the particular forms of his finitude, are largely self-generated. 'What if [the treatment] stops working?' he types, with shaking hands, daring prognosis to turn uncertainty into despair rather than into hope. Doubt is a fearful form of finitude if it is unreasoned and self-fulfilling.

There is also the finitude of our *spectating* – our judging, enjoying, waiting and suffering. We are subject to finitude in them all, and that finitude is even merciful in some respects: it puts a limit upon suffering, such that the very things (the reality and symptoms of physical and mental frailty) that remind us of our finitude also constitute it and, in the end, relieve us through bringing it fully upon us.

And, painfully, there is the finitude of our *separation*. We are of course social creatures – doubtless irreducibly so in language as well as in conduct[6] – and yet we are still the individual loci of our own experiences of a notionally shared world. Hence the importance of both the fact, and the fragility, of our attempts to capture, express and convey our first-person experiences so that we are confident of being understood and recognised for who we are: whether we are falling in love, accounting for misdeeds or seeking support on the illness-journey. We continually 'frame' the world from a perspective that, at the time, no one else can precisely occupy. The frame itself is a form (and indeed an archetype) of finitude, never precisely aligned with any other frame. Metaphors can enliven our descriptions, but they succeed only if they are grasped in something like the way we ourselves coined them. (And what is our criterion for knowing when *that* has happened? Merely prosaic agreement will never quite suffice.) We hope that what we say connects sufficiently well with another's experience for them to recognise that experience – or something like it – in us. A prognosis informed by shared experience may be no more certain than one that is not, but it may have additional resonance for the patient looking ahead at the very same uncertainties. We are meaning-making creatures and we try – perhaps because we need to try – to make some kind of meaning out of every experience. But we can be no more confident that others grasp the meanings that we make than we can be confident of grasping theirs, and that is a sobering thought.

Most obviously of all, perhaps, is the finitude of our *knowing*. Prognosis, both a defiance of uncertainty and an attempt to map how far the future is open, perfectly exemplifies this finitude even in defying it. It may be true that 'we know more than we can tell',[7] but it is also true that we know less than can be told. This is true in what I might call a 'domestic' sense, in the ordinary recognition that we cannot know beyond what we (or, via report, others) happen to have experienced. But it is true also in, for want of a better term, a more existential sense. The conditions under which it is possible for human experience to come about and be sustained, the general circumstances of our nature and the material reality we inhabit, are opaque to us. Too large, perhaps too terrifying, to do normal business with, such circumstances must be relegated to poetic and philosophical speculation in order that the ordinary conduct of ordinary life and ordinary illness and death may proceed. But given a moment's respite from the routine, we sometimes sense that something is needed to lend meaning to the otherwise preposterous accident of human experience arising unbidden in a once-sterile material universe. Rachel's having the child that she is determined to carry to term will challenge her management of her diabetes (amid much else, as every parent knows), and we do not know whether she will succeed. Liz, more timidly, contemplates pregnancy in the improbable company of an Internet forum – a near-perfect metaphor for our age of uncertainty. She will search in vain online for the prognosis she really wants, since her self-doubts have had longer to mature and they go deeper than her epilepsy. But even so, what is true for Rachel can be true for Liz, too: bringing into the world a new life is a peerlessly vivid – in all senses – route to defying finitude, for a time.

Prognosis, by reminding us of our fleshly finitude, reminds us too of our existential finitude. Thus it sharpens our need to know that there may be something beyond or behind our existence (or at least our need to believe in it) – a need that is, of necessity, 'unconsummated' in ordinary life. Especially when a prognosis is unfavourable or grave, it sharpens our similarly 'unconsummated' desire to *transcend* our circumstances. Perhaps it is above all in this sense that prognosis as fore-knowing is a kind of defiance of finitude. In his *Summer Meditations* Vaclav Havel suggests that it is actually rational, and intrinsic to human experience, to hope that there is more to life, and hence to reality, than the world of experience as we know it.[8] If this be true in general, how much more true is it when either natural age or prognosis in serious illness paints the nearness of approaching finitude? As Raymond Tallis puts it:

The sense of finitude animates a desperate desire to make a deeper, more coherent, sense of things, to seize hold of it in its greatness, to be equal in consciousness to the great world on which we find ourselves, of which we are conscious in a piecemeal, sequential, fragmented, small-world way. The idea of death is a threat, a goad, and an inspiration. And its power is available to all of us who aim to live abundantly.[9]

III – THE IDEA OF THE NOUMENAL

Recently I sat on a park bench in the sunshine in the otherwise almost deserted college grounds where I work, rued my torpid middle age (and the bones that no longer clamour for physical challenge but are disappointingly contented by the prospect of inactivity) and settled down to watch a tiny beetle crawling laboriously up a twig, over the edge of a leaf and along the leaf's underside. It occurred to me that had I time, patience and refreshment, and were I to sit and watch for long enough, I might plausibly witness such a creature's entire course of birth, life and death, and observe its every action – with little understanding on my part, of course, but with a certain existential sympathy that would outlive its six-legged object. Compared to my own consciousness, the beetle's consciousness is not only more limited but vastly more fleeting. Such an ephemeral 'consciousness' would arise and disappear, vanishing *forever* in any subjective sense (if we can speak of a subject here): vanishing as though it had never been, its only continued validation subsisting in the mind and continuing consciousness of the watcher.

But, in the long run, it is the same for us, too. One day our consciousness will be as though it had never been, for all that our deeds may outlive us: only the consciousnesses of those who survive us will validate the claim that behind our deeds lay not automata but thinking, experiencing, willing subjects as well.

Bizarrely, we can glimpse this for ourselves at first hand in special circumstances, of which an example known to me personally produces what I will call the 'midazolam problem'. Midazolam, a sedative/hypnotic from the benzodiazepine group of drugs, is notorious as Rohypnol, the 'date-rape drug,' for its memory-suppressant effect. Fortunately that very effect, so despicably used in sexual assault, is in other contexts therapeutically valuable. In particular it is invaluable in helping patients to endure unpleasant procedures that require from them sufficient consciousness as to be able to cooperate with the clinicians. Now I use the word 'endure' but this is problematic: for to endure something is, among other things, to experience it, and an important question arises over the status of *experience* in regard to any portion of conscious life of which no subjective trace remains. This is important in thinking about death, for in death, so far as we can tell, all subjective traces are removed of not just a portion but the entirety of a given conscious life.

A personal clinical anecdote may bring out what is at stake. I was a few years ago obliged to have my insides explored by an endoscope (a flexible and steerable optical tube inserted into the body). It is a procedure that no one could relish, but unfortunately it is one that requires an aware patient to respond to instructions, and hence is incompatible with anaesthesia in the ordinary sense. Pain-relieving drugs may also be offered as an adjunct, but sedation and amnesia are the primary comforts aimed at through midazolam.

My encounter with this much-feared procedure, once I had somehow dragged my shivering green-gowned self onto the operating table, was in the event an entirely untroubled one, although baffling. The ensuing experience consisted wholly of conversation *and nothing else*: lying on the table, I asked the surgeon whether he had administered the sedative sufficiently early for it to take full effect, and he replied that he certainly had, for it was being delivered intravenously. A nurse then *immediately* asked me whether I would like tea or coffee with my biscuit. I politely pointed out that this seemed very premature, and she politely rejoined that it was nothing of the kind since I was in the post-operative recovery room. And, unbelievably, I was – with the endoscopy apparently completed. (Moreover, within half an hour my wife and I were in a restaurant enjoying a hearty lunch.) Somehow this absurd suturing of a gash in time struck me in the moment of re-arousal as being amusing rather than shocking, and it took a little while for the philosopher in me to creep out from his trauma-evading refuge.

I have since thought long and hard about what one can say of such a seamless 'book-ended' gap in life – an 'experiectomy', as one might call it surgically. Subjectively, the inaccessibility to me of anything that happened while I was sedated is total, full-stop. Anything that I may have appeared to experience, to participate in, to respond to, while under sedation is now, and (I am convinced) was then, an appearance only for others, in their memory and in whatever other traces may persist of those events. Events are not in themselves experiences. Responses and behaviours are not in themselves experiences. My memories of what happened under sedation have not so much been washed away: rather they were never laid down. And this complete inaccessibility of 'what happened' seems to me to be radical and significant. For me, subjectively, 'what happened' is now either a mere third-person report – as though of an event not involving me, and that I never witnessed – or it is *annihilated*, inasmuch as it was void from the outset. No continuing *me* was there to validate it. The only *me* involved is so completely sliced-off from the *me* of events before and since, that it may as well never have existed; indeed in no accessible sense did it ever exist. The sedation marks a perfect absence from the continuity of *me* – so thoroughly absent, so thoroughly without subjective validation, that what 'happened' under sedation never happened.

It seems to me that death is like that with regard to the temporary bubble of conscious experience that we presently inhabit. Our traces will, for a while, constitute events remembered by, or later reported to, others, but that is all. In the vast eternity of darkness, experience flickers briefly: and during the flickering we can realise and articulate this conundrum, but we will be extinguished and the interruption to the darkness will be so completely annulled that it will be as if the flickering never happened. Indeed if *all* other flickerings – each capable to a small extent of recording and recalling the fact of neighbouring, overlapping flickerings of others – came to an end (and why should they not? Why should the phenomenon of organic consciousness persist indefinitely?) then its having happened will be indistinguishable from its not having happened. The distinction will have no meaning.

I realise how pessimistic, how nihilistic, this sounds but it is not meant like that. I am not lamenting any of it; I am merely recognising it in that minor herald of individual annihilation that I met in my temporary self-interruption by midazolam. Death finds only a poor metaphor in sleep, as Fingarette has pointed out[10]: but it seems to me that in chemical oblivion it finds a genuinely powerful one. That procedure's importance lies in presenting to anyone who has undergone it *without leaving any experiential trace*, as in my own case, a vivid illustration of what the annihilation of experience actually means. Whatever 'happened' to me, however I responded (was 'I' brave? Did 'I' cry out in pain or distress? Could the surgeon secure 'my' cooperation?) 'happened' in no enduring sense except in the acts and the recollections of those around. The only guarantor of the events in question is the consciousnesses of others who were there; the 'I' who was there, *if* indeed 'he' ever existed in any sense other than a purely behavioural one, was obliterated.

Thus the ephemeral nature of my own conscious experience is made vivid and acute for me – without sadness or regret, but certainly as an object of wonder. So long as I am alive and conscious I can continue to assure and validate the reality of my subjective existence; but if there was a time before my conscious life and if there will be a time after it, it is assured and validated only in the consciousnesses of others. Hence, perhaps, our desire to think that a consciousness larger than our own could solve the problem of our own ephemeral nature. As individuals, we like to think that in some attenuated sense we can exert our presence, even our will, beyond our material existence – in the memories of others and in the carrying out of our wishes, in the funeral rites and the reading and execution of our wills, in our letters and writings and in any other traces that we may leave and that may have influence on the lives of others after us. Of course the consciousness of a collective of others who are like us, and whose memories embrace us, is not always enough for us. Indeed, unless entropy can be indefinitely postponed, collective consciousness and shared memories will in the long run not be a sufficient guarantor of *anyone's* ever having existed as a subjective reality. So some people imagine God, whose omni-consciousness covers every gap, now and always. Others imagine something else, through a kind of personification in art, philosophy, books and music, although these too would in the long run need an imprint on some eternal realm. At any rate it seems that it is the imagination that is our present refuge from finitude – an existential prognosis of the most speculative and supplicant kind.

Of course even in writing this I am to some extent imagining here. Perhaps – even in philosophical conjecture – we are all compelled to imagine. Perhaps imagination is a condition of learning, which in turn requires our mastering the prognostic as well as descriptive and retrospective roles of language, grasping that what is properly said now can also properly be said, in the right circumstances, in the future. As Wittgenstein realised, we are marked out as language users proper when we can learn and take hold of the meaning, the coherent possibility, of the intensely prognostic phrase 'and so on'.[11] Often we appeal to the imagination to offer a glimpse beyond what we can know. Prognosis, too, is an act of imagination – a projection beyond what we immediately know, but based upon what we (and others) have known. It challenges a contingent type of finitude – we happen not yet to have seen where an illness is going to lead, but if we wait patiently we will do so, and the moving curtain that clarifies the extent of our finitude will roll onward a little way.

But what of a projection beyond all that we could ever know, and based upon nothing we have ever known but merely upon the fact that we can know anything at all: a projection challenging a finitude that is total? Such conjectures, articulated or not, hover around us when we contemplate death as the only certainty in a future that is otherwise more or less open, depending upon the nature and confidence of our prognosis. The thought of complete finitude tempts us to suppose that something unknown, unseen, underlies the existence that is ours and with which we suppose we are familiar. We yearn to connect with something that will transcend our finitude, something whose power as Larkin put it 'outbuilds cathedrals';[12] and if we cannot connect with it we nonetheless yearn to posit it and give it a name.

In fact this yearning is not without philosophical support. Kant[13] and, later, Schopenhauer[14] breathtakingly realised that since we know the world only through experience, the spatial and temporal and causal forms taken by that experience are a feature of our minds, not of the world itself independently of us. (As they appreciated, space, time and causation are the conditions of our experience and are found only where experience is found: that is, subjectively. See Magee for a beautifully accessible explanation of their thought.[15,16]) Necessarily, we cannot experience the formative processes and constraints themselves, only their consequences.

Equally our daily experience of our own free will discloses an aspect of our own nature that can never itself be part of the empirical world described by science – there is no experience, no part of the observable world, that is 'the willing' or 'the deciding' to do something. We know that we *do* will and decide, but we cannot catch ourselves willing or deciding; all we can know are their observable consequences in the world describable by science. The world is, in short, only partially revealed to us in experience. Some part of it underlies that experience and, in underlying it, is beyond all possibility of being itself experienced. Astonishingly, we ourselves, as willing agents capable of acting in the world, simultaneously inhabit both the empirical world of science and the larger reality that underlies the empirical world yet is not itself bounded by space, time or causal connection. That larger reality must be there – logically must – but we can never know it directly, although we can reason our way towards acknowledging it.

In close (although not identical) progression of thought, Kant and Schopenhauer called this unknown the *noumenal*; although neither of them associated it with any kind of personal existence, the noumenal occupies a philosophical place that somewhat recalls the idea of an eternal realm familiar in religious thought, a realm that in some sense answers to our yearning for there to be something that transcends our own finitude. (The noumenal, incidentally, offers neither proof nor disproof of God's existence.) We may or may not take comfort from the answer; notoriously, Schopenhauer himself did not. But if we do take comfort from it, that comfort is supported by philosophical reasons to regard the idea of the noumenal as logically more compelling than mere psychological palliation.

Somehow as we get older, or as we brush more closely against illnesses that could one day be serious, we become more conscious of our finitude; we have more reason to wonder whether that finitude is total; and we become more conscious that the story of existence is our story, too, and not simply the story of those choirs of the dead who have preceded us. And this is a consequence not merely of serious prognosis: *any* prognosis, even a happy one, is nonetheless a reminder of the continuity of our fleshly frailty and vulnerability; we are, after all, born with an indeterminate sentence of death. When we reflect on this, the conjecture that reality may be somehow veiled starts to haunt us – whether we believe on the one hand that, on lifting a corner of the veil, we will glimpse the noumenal or, on the other, that we will confront nothing more than 'the solving emptiness that lies beneath'.[5]

IV – A CODA: ECHOES IN MUSIC

In this chapter prognosis, the medical act, has fallen into the role of flag-bearer for how we look at, and face, future uncertainties of other kinds: our finitude is guaranteed by our mortal nature, even while it is defied by our imaginations, so it is natural for medical prognosis to become almost a metonym for looking forward in an existential sense.

Lakoff and Johnson, in their celebrated and now-classic study *Metaphors We Live By*,[17] envisage the linguistic inevitability of structuring our depictions of the world around a framework of metaphor largely rooted in physical, spatial, experience. The level(!) on which metaphors operate(!) determines their visibility(!) (to use three more metaphors). The metaphorical uses of orientational terms such as 'up' and 'down' to refer to changes of extent, value, frequency, volume, intensity and so forth are so embedded (metaphor again) as virtually to merge (and again!) into the literal: they are simply unavoidable. But we can use metaphors and tropes more consciously than this, and sometimes we do so when literal descriptions are either dry to the point of futility, or imaginatively inaccessible. In our first Volume in this series, I drew on music and musicality as metaphors for the ordinary conduct of a modestly flourishing life.[18] The ready availability of musical metaphors in many aspects of lived experience rests in part on the intense relationship between musical experience and embodiment (something that Mark Johnson draws out in some detail,[19] true to his general grounding of metaphor in physical experience). I would like to return briefly to music-as-metaphor now in closing these remarks on prognosis.

But first, a prefatory note. Music's rich metaphorical resources have long been recognised, seized-upon, exploited and cultivated: rhythm, harmony and melody all lend themselves readily to the task of characterising both what life is and what it might be, and in contexts ranging from the banalities of greeting-card doggerel to the rarefied nuances of cultural history,[2] as well as to the small change of lived experience (witness Anne Macleod's memorable characterisation of Jen's last hours 'fighting that rasping symphony of failing breath'). In my own case I find music almost to outgrow its metaphorical role; to become at times almost the dominant partner, such that life's events take on for me a quasi-musical form – life's rhythms and developments and exigencies becoming forms of expression, among many other alternative forms, of musical possibility. Indeed – however strange it may seem when written down – I find it difficult to shake off the conviction that life, human-ness, human embodiment, are themselves forms of musicality amid the endless musical variety of the material Universe. (In partial defence, related convictions explosively animated some important philosophical reaction to the emergence of 'absolute' music in the nineteenth century, in the writings of Schelling, Schopenhauer, Nietzsche and Novalis among others.[2]) At any rate, it was in this spirit that I tried to convey the experience of serious illness in Volume 1, and try now to offer a few figurative thoughts on futures and finitude.

First, I have noted more than once that the idea of prognosis – *forward looking* – reminds us of our mortality even when a given prognosis is friendly.

Our declining years, in an ordinary life-span and given averagely satisfactory health, mark an autumnal period that can be thought of as either a cadence to a theme, or as the coda to that musical movement in which our life more largely consists. In our maturity we may expect to have become settled to the point of predictability in identity and purposes, habits and beliefs. Thus we depart from the settled notation of our lives either by way of a temporary, improvisatory diversion, a riff; or more extendedly, discovering or experimenting with previously unsuspected ideas and goals. New stories may emerge, unexpected insights and blossoming (although it is also true that, in improvisation, themes can also dreadfully unravel, before we realise it or can respond).

Prognosis implies neither definite ending nor definite limitation – it does not 'wrap life up' as Jane Macnaughton has pointed out – and we are normally able to keep open the possibility of new branchings, new ways of flourishing, even in our last years. A musical coda can be improvisatory; it does not, or at least need not, settle finally and fixedly the fate of the music's *motifs*. From Beethoven's innovations onward (fully half of the fourth movement of his Eighth Symphony is devoted to an extended and exploratory coda), the great symphonists would often experiment as much in a coda as in that same movement's 'official' development section, and there is something infinitely rich about both musical and biographical subject matter that defies the expectation of ordered closure that a coda, even a long coda, ordinarily brings. A coda can be a variation upon an existing theme within our lives; occasionally it can, almost experimentally, introduce new and wholly unexpected material. In music this is difficult to do convincingly; perhaps it is difficult in life, too – here, it may even be made possible by the provocation of an unexpected prognosis, bringing the resources of a resolve to make the most of a lifespan that turns out to be foreseeably shorter than one had hoped.

Now music relies on the openness of the future, and in a way that is almost playful. The structures of repetition and rhythm, and of established consonance and harmony, provide the stable backdrop across which melody is drawn out. At the most basic level of listening, melody's capacity to satisfy us, no less than its capacity to surprise us, relies upon our anticipating its direction ('co-composing' as we listen[20]) and having our expectations fulfilled or evaded as the case may be.

Curiously, even repeated listenings, even to music that we know well, retain a reference to – or, better, a reliance upon – an open future. This is not simply because different performances or interpretations of the same work can produce substantially distinct listening experiences, but (I think, more fundamentally) because 'the same' music is always what it is against the backdrop of unnumbered alternative possible pathways through the same marvellous matrix of other possible harmonies, melodies and rhythmic complexities. Western diatonic music has been exploited abundantly for more than four centuries and yet it is still capable of new possibilities; an obituary for the late Benjamin Britten praised him for his capacity to write original tunes 'in C major' (standing for music's most well-ploughed furrow); Jason Robert Brown's contemporary musical *The Last Five Years* is musically fresh and inventive within a harmonic vocabulary that would still have been found recognisable by Bach and comfortable by Schumann. Music continually suggests the re-opening of the future.

But music is not boundlessly open (indeed it has even been suggested, apocryphally, that 'All great music is inevitable'). In this sense music relies also upon important finitudes – those necessary for the stability of recognisable forms, genres and traditions, and necessary for the boundaries and framing that are entailed by the very notion of structure, musical or otherwise. Complex structures such as sonata form rely on future expectations that are partially bounded because we know in advance the general sort of things that we should expect if the music is to count as sonata form. Not boundlessly open, then – yet still substantially open because there are indefinitely many different ways in which those expectations can be met, or flouted. Indeed one of the most satisfying moments in a sonata-form movement, the arrival of the recapitulation after the development section, is psychologically powerful to the extent that we are both prepared for it and yet surprised by it.

It is also crucially true that music begins and ends in silence (as, presumably, does conscious life) and this 'framing' silence marks the very finitude that gives a piece of music its identity, let alone its value. I suspect that the idea of unending music would be meaningless or at best pointless; music's finitude is essential to its having, in the case of any given piece of music, either direction or completeness. One is tempted to feel that this is true of a life, too – whether it be one that flourished or one that languished. We cannot really imagine what an unbounded life could mean; still less can we imagine living it.

Spitzer reminds us that melody was for Nietzsche 'primary and universal'; that Novalis conceived the soul as 'acoustic'.[21] But in noting that Schopenhauer saw melody as 'linking man and nature' he seriously understates the case. Schopenhauer, as Magee makes clear, regarded music as

> a direct manifestation of the noumenal. Just as the phenomenal [familiar, material] world is the self-manifestation of the noumenal in experience, so is music. It is the voice of the metaphysical will.[22]

It is perhaps tempting to dismiss this as meaningless, as bizarre, or as unmanageably obscure. Schopenhauer himself knew that he was condemned to use language somewhat figuratively. I have already admitted that music's relation to life is for me more than metaphorical – or that the metaphor's direction does not lead necessarily from music to life, but rather that life sometimes seems to me to be an instance of music's possibilities. On first hearing, at the age of 54 years, the opening bars of Bach's 'St Anne' Prelude for organ I realised that all of the elements of diatonic music, which have for my whole life been the constituents of my inmost strainings and struggles, my regalings and revelries, were being properly disclosed, announced, to me for the first time. It was as if light had *de novo* fallen upon an open book, in which the workings of an ordered Universe were vouchsafed. There was nothing personal in this – in that sense this was no individual prognosis. And our individual finitude – a fleeting spark of awareness-of-being, wholly adventitious in a material Universe, validated by nothing, un-extendable, ultimately un-shareable – was no less incomprehensible or absurd. The absurdity seemed, however, less important. The future was indeed open, its terms drawn in musical possibility.

REFERENCES

1. Fingarette H. *Death: philosophical Soundings*. Peru, ILL: Carus Publishing; 1996. p. 57.
2. Wackenroder quoted in Spitzer M. *Metaphor and Musical Thought*. Chicago, CA: University of Chicago Press; 2004. p. 281.
3. Papineau D. Methodology: the elements of the philosophy of science. In: Grayling A.C., editor. *Philosophy: a guide through the subject*. Oxford: Oxford University Press; 1995. pp. 123–80.
4. Holland A. A fortnight in my life is missing: reflections on the status of the human 'pre-embryo'. *Journal of Applied Philosophy*. 1990; 7: 25–37.
5. Larkin P. Ambulances: *The Whitsun weddings*. London: Faber and Faber; 1964.
6. Wittgenstein L. *Philosophical Investigations*. Oxford: Basil Blackwell; 1958.
7. Polanyi M. *The Tacit Dimension*. New York, NY: Anchor Books; 1967.
8. Havel V. *Summer Meditations*. New York, NY: Alfred A. Knopf; 1992.
9. Tallis R. *In Defence Of Wonder and Other Philosophical Reflections*. Durham: Acumen Publishing; 2012. p. 211.
10. Fingarette H. *Death: philosophical Soundings*. Peru, ILL: Carus Publishing; 1996. p. 19.
11. Wittgenstein L. *Philosophical Investigations*. Oxford: Basil Blackwell; 1958. Sections 201ff.
12. Larkin P. The building. In: *High Windows*. London: Faber & Faber; 1974.
13. Kant I. *A Critique Of Pure Reason*. London: Macmillan; 1929.
14. Schopenhauer A. *The World As Will and Representation*. New York, NY: Dover Books; 1966.
15. Magee B. *Confessions Of a Philosopher*. London: Weidenfeld & Nicholson; 1997.
16. Magee B. *The Philosophy Of Schopenhauer*. Oxford: Oxford University Press; 1983.
17. Lakoff G., Johnson M. *Metaphors We Live By*. Chicago, CA: University of Chicago Press; 1980.
18. Evans H.M. Music, interrupted: an illness observed from within. In: Evans H.M., Ahlzen. R., Heath, I., editors. *Medical Humanities Companion Volume One: symptom*. Oxford: Radcliffe Publishing; 2008. pp. 14–26.
19. Johnson M. *The Meaning Of the Body*. Chicago, CA: University of Chicago Press; 2007.
20. Evans H.M. *Listening To Music*. London: Macmillan; 1990.
21. Wackenroder quoted in Spitzer M. *Metaphor and Musical Thought*. Chicago, CA: University of Chicago Press; 2004. pp. 282–3.
22. Magee B. *Confessions Of a Philosopher*. London: Weidenfeld & Nicholson; 1997. pp. 503–4.

Postscript

In about the 17th century, the word 'genius' assumed the meaning that we recognise today, that is a person of significant intellectual capacity. However, it has an older meaning – that of 'a guardian spirit' – that also persists to this day. The word is derived from the Latin *gignere* (to give birth, to bring forth, to bear). Our genius in the *Companion* series is a person of great intellectual capacity *and* a guardian spirit who helped to bring forth the four volumes in the *Medical Humanities Companion* series. Anne McLeod, through the paradoxical authenticity of fiction, has introduced us to the 'real' people around whom each volume in the series has been built. Anne's insights as a clinician combined with her skill as a storyteller have brought Rachel, Jake, Liz, Jen and Geoff to life.

We close with one last look at how their lives go on. In the postscripts that Anne has provided, each character is trying to communicate something – through a diary entry, an anonymous questionnaire, an Internet post or a letter. Each character has been, from time to time, in communication with their doctor, but the doctors have been busy and preoccupied, working under the pressure of an underfunded healthcare system, with limited opportunities to fully understand what each character most wants to communicate.

Each character expresses the need for a close confidante, someone whom they can trust. But this is an increasingly estranged world, where fewer and fewer people are close to one another. A recent United Nations (UN) report notes that:

> The 20th Century has witnessed remarkable changes in family structures and dynamics in Western Europe and North America: smaller household sizes, a further shift from extended to nuclear families, a decrease in nuptiality and an increase in separation or divorce.[1]

Iona Heath touched on this problem in Chapter 9, quoting Arthur Kleinman's reflection that 'few of the tragedies at life's end are as rending to the clinician as that of the frail elderly patient who has no one to tell the life story to'. This is the long-term prognosis for a society in which families are small, children are scattered and work takes precedence over family life.

Rachel needed someone to hear her story instead of endlessly 'educating' her; Jake lives with the regret that he was never able to tell his story to the one person who understood – his first girlfriend, Carol. Liz, as a single parent, has hardly ever had time to think about her own needs, and only now is she beginning to construct a new story – a story that she would be confident to tell. Jen and Geoff told their stories to one another until illness drew them apart, instead of bringing them together. In every case, the lines of communication are imperilled.

When will we learn?

Rudolf Virchov saw in medicine a potential yet to be realised. He wrote:

> Should medicine ever fulfil its great ends, it must enter into the larger political and social life of our time; it must indicate the barriers which obstruct the normal completion of the life cycle and remove them. Should it ever come to pass, Medicine, whatever it may then be, will become the common good of all.[2]

1. Cliquet R. *Major Trends Affecting Families In the New Millennium: Western Europe and North America*; 2003. www.un.org/esa/socdev/family/Publications/mtcliquet.pdf (accessed 20 April 2013).
2. Virchov cited in Ackerkrecht EH. *Rudolf Virchow*. Madison, WI: University of Wisconsin Press; 1953. p. 126.

Postscript Stories

RACHEL: 15 YEARS OLD

Diary

I never told no one about missing. Well, they never asked, did they? It's: You're not doing this and you're not doing that. *How* much insulin? *When?* No one asks if you're regular, if Aunt Flo is visiting.

Knocked up. Like the film. LOL.

But I won't be having no abortion. Mum is standing by me. Never thought she'd be that cool.

The hospital today was OK, though. At least, the nurses were fine. The doctor went on and on. Diabetes. Education. Like they do. I hate that stuff.

Still, maybe I'll get my own place. A flat? :)

JAKE: 30 YEARS OLD

Quality of life: additional comments

Jake's pen hovers over the blank box on the survey sheet. Finally, it moves, the words forming, flowing.

Additional comments. Eh?

Psoriasis has ruined my life. It has wasted weeks – no, months – of work-time. I spend longer in waiting rooms each year than most folk do in Tenerife. I've met all kinds of medics – the good, the not so good – and all kinds of nurses, too. None of them has ever been able to offer what I really want, which is not to have psoriasis.

Never to have had it.

This last treatment is best so far, but what about the future?

What if it stops working?

His hand lingers above that last sentence, shaking.

LIZ: 38 YEARS OLD

Posted on Mumsnet

Hopeful 10 April 2012 on Thursday 5 April at 18:02:51.

I'm thinking about a pregnancy, and wonder if anyone else may be in a similar position.

I've had two episodes of LLETZ, one for CIN2 and one for CIN1. I'm 38 and also on Valproate (for another condition). The doctors have been great, and I have an appointment at a pre-conception clinic, but if you've been in my position, I'd love to hear from you.

JEN AND GEOFF

Letter from Jane to Geoff's daughter Mary

Dear Mary,

I was up at the hospital today to see your father. He's in a bad way. Flat on his back. Stares past you. Recognises no one. Of course, he's not been in the real world for a while.

The charge nurse called me over for a chat. I hadn't realised that you'd been phoning every week. I'm glad that you've been in touch with them, Mary, but is it really wise to be laying down the law? Those drugs you insisted they give him for his raised blood fats just gave him a skin rash. And for you to demand they do everything possible to bring him back if he were to collapse – have you seen them do resuscitation, Mary? I mean, not just on the telly? Why would you want them to do that? What on this earth is there to bring him back to? I know you love your dad but, Mary, come and see him. You'd understand better if you did.

We've not always seen eye to eye, I know. Truth to tell, I was just as angry as you when he got together with Jen. But, Mary, it's not for you or me to judge. That was all a long time ago. Geoff is suffering. The doctors and the nurses have done what they can. Enough's enough.

Come and see him, Mary. Let nature take its course.

Yours affectionately,

Aunt Jane

Index

absenteeism
  and medical labelling 85
acupuncture
  sham 22
adaptation to 'illness
  and 'becoming' xiii, 53, 56, 57–8, 59
ADHD (attention deficit hyperactivity
    disorder) 84
ageing population 94
ageing, technology and death 93–101
  and the 'fair innings' argument 98–100
  and medicine as a commodity 96–7
  and technological activism 94–6
alcoholism 80
ALS (amyotrophic lateral sclerosis) 57
Alzheimer's disease 44, 45
American Psychiatric Association 84–5
  DSM (Diagnostic and Statistical Manual)
    84–5
amniocentesis 86
amyotrophic lateral sclerosis (ALS) 57
Anglo-American medical ideology
  and healthism 83
animal magnetism theory 73
anti-depressants 84
anxiety
  and prognostication 16
Aristotle 45
asthma
  and sham acupuncture 22
atherosclerosis 21
Athill, Diana
  Somewhere Towards the End 64, 99,
    102
  Yesterday Morning 93
attention deficit hyperactivity disorder
    (ADHD) 84
autoimmune diseases
  and prognosis-as-lived 18, 20
  prognostication 17
autonomy
  and chronic illness 48
  harm caused by 79
  and healthism 82

  and instrumental reason 86
  respect for xii
  versus individualism 87–9

Bach Flower Remedies 74
Bach, Johann Sebastian 119
  'St Anne' Prelude for organ 120
basal cell carcinoma (BCC) 9–10
Batmanghelidj, Dr Fereydoon 74
Beauchamp, TL xii
Beckett, Samuel
  Malone Dies 94–5
becoming xiii, 53–64
  and change over time 53, 55–6, 62, 64
  and choice 53, 61–3
  and disruption 56–61
  flourishing in xiii, 63–4
  and inability 54–5
Beethoven, Ludwig van 118
being
  finitude of our 109–10
  and time 28
beneficence
  as the task of the doctor xii
benign prophecies 76
Berger, John 16
bioethics
  and individual autonomy 89
biological processes
  and prognosis-as-lived 19–20
biomedical parameters
  and prognostication 21
biomedical research
  and instrumental reason 86
  regulation of 79, 89–90
biopsychosocial perspective on prognosis
    31–2
  patient's story 35–6
biotechnology
  and medicalisation 84
bipolar disorder 20
Blair, Tony
  A Journey 45
Bloom, Arnold 51

CPD with Radcliffe

You can now use a selection of our books to achieve CPD (Continuing Professional Development) points through directed reading.

We provide a free online form and downloadable certificate for your appraisal portfolio. Look for the CPD logo and register with us at: **www.radcliffehealth.com/cpd**

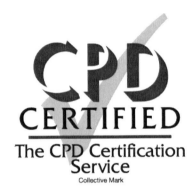